Living with Cancer

(Stage 4 - and never giving up)

Andy Partington

Photography : Charlie R

Thank You 1

The Moment of Truth.............................3

Bucket List Frenzy.................................5

The Real Book..7

The Shift 10

Why This Book Really Exists...................11

The Promises 12

Before We Go Any Further 14

Jim Legging It...17

Home Sweet Home 24

11 Morar Drive.......................................26

Academia 35

The Road To Somewhere.......................40

New Town, New Schools 46

Time To Grow Up 52

Christopher John Riley...........................63

The Why 65

High Flying 69

A Career Change....................................73

Blast From The Past...............................78

In Trouble Again 83

Croeso I Gymru 94

Should I Stay or Should I Go?................97

Valbonne, Bridgend................................102

Dream Dream Dream...............................105

DIY and NJP - The Sequel 109

Paul's Casino..115

Heaven or Hell..119

Betrayal 125

Back In The Car Trade.............................130

Time To Go Home 134

The Prodigal Son Returns 138

The Queensway 143

An English Country Garden.....................148

Perth, WA - Part 1 152

Perth, WA - Part 2 156

Wedded Bliss 160

Zena's Prophetic Words 163

Man Utd 3 - Chelsea 1 170

You're Kidding, Right? 175

Please Come Home 180

Hailstones and Other Madness...............183

The Road To Nowhere 188

The Northern Territory 194

Trailer Trashed 198

Rain, Rain, and More Bloody Rain 203

Bye Bye Cairns, Hello WA 207

Old Blighty 212

Back To Reality 218

The End of an Era 224

Health Problems 227

Back At The Quacks 233

Plans and Promises 245

Going It Alone 250

One Day At A Time 253

Shopping For A New Life 255

Rebuilding More Than Myself 257

On The Up 259

Chemo 262

Side Effects 265

The Darkest Side Effect 268

Round Two 271

The Diet 277

Radiotherapy...288

The Bell 293

The Letter 297

Post Treatment 302

Write A Book 321

What's Next?...334

Epilogue 339

Acknowledgements - The Roll Call Of
Legends 341

Reader Q&A – You Asked, I Definitely Made
Up the Answers.....................................343

About The Author 344

"Laughter is the best medicine"

....Origin Unknown

Thank You

Thank you for choosing to read this book. I wonder what brought you here. Perhaps you – or someone you care about – has recently received a cancer diagnosis. If that's the case, I want to be upfront: this isn't a deep dive into the science of cancer. If you're looking for medical jargon or cutting-edge research, I'm afraid this book will disappoint. And I'm truly sorry for that.

When I was diagnosed four years ago, I felt completely overwhelmed – not just by the news, but by how little I understood about what was happening inside my own body. Since then, I haven't tried to master every microscopic detail of cancer, but I've learned enough to make informed decisions about my care. I didn't dive into the science because, quite frankly, that's not where my strengths lie. My oncologists–with their years of training – have handled that side brilliantly. The last thing they need is me weighing in with medical knowledge which barely extends beyond applying a Band-Aid.

So I focused on the one thing I *could* influence: how I live my life. This book is about that journey – the choices I've made, the changes I've embraced, and the ways I've tried to reclaim the time I have left and make it meaningful. I wanted to take back some control. Not by mastering oncology textbooks, but by reshaping my everyday life in ways which brought me peace, comfort, and purpose.

I don't claim to have the answers – not even one of

them. But if sharing my story helps even one person find hope, clarity, or courage in the face of their own diagnosis, then every word I've written will have been worth it.

This book isn't just about enduring cancer. It's about *living* – boldly, messily, with heart, humour, and a refusal to let fear call the shots. If that message resonates with you, then we're already connected in a way words can't describe.

The Moment of Truth

2 p.m., July 23rd, 2020. While COVID was rampaging around the globe and everyone was panic-buying toilet paper, baking banana bread, or plunging headlong into conspiracy theories, I was sitting opposite an oncologist who, in turn, was sitting behind a desk large enough to land a light aircraft on.

That's when I heard the words no man ever wants to hear:

I had prostate cancer.

But not the "snip it out, talk about some pelvic floor exercises and move on" kind. Oh no. This ambitious little bastard had gone on a world tour. It had packed its bags and caught a flight to the lymph nodes in my lower abdomen. Stage four. Incurable. Irreversible. Irrefutably shit!

"Oh," I replied casually, as though he'd just informed me my Netflix subscription had expired.

Still, it doesn't sound so bad if you say it quickly.

Oddly, there was a silver lining – and I clung to it like it was the last Tim Tam in the packet. Medicare, bless its bureaucratic heart, would do what it could. They couldn't cure me, but they'd take a red-hot go at slowing things down and giving me a bit more time. I was grateful. And terrified.

Naturally, I asked *the* question – the one we all rehearse in our heads and hope never to say aloud.

"How long have I got, Doc?"

He looked at me, calm as you like, and said, "At least two years."

At that moment, July 23rd officially overtook every bad birthday, and dental appointment, to become the worst day of my life.

But hey – we'll return to this point in time later in the book. Assuming I live long enough to write it. (lol)

Bucket List Frenzy

Three days.

That's how long it took after receiving the news before I began planning to skydive from the International Space Station, learn competitive salsa dancing without looking like I'd been tasered, and – oh yes – write a book.

Why? Because when your world flips upside down like a drunken trapeze act, the only logical thing to do is panic... then panic some more... then make a list.

Yes, a bucket list. One of those "before I cark it" catalogues of grand adventures and life-affirming moments, usually scribbled by people in midlife crisis mode or whilst getting stuck into their third glass of merlot. Except this wasn't midlife. This could very well be *end of life*. So I thought, *"To hell with it. Bring on the skydiving, the salsa, and the self-discovery – and I'll throw in a llama trek through Peru while I'm at it."*

The idea came to me at 2:47 a.m. – because that's when all good existential clarity hits. I lay in bed, having a full-on stare-down with the ceiling fan, picturing the Angel of Death peeking from behind the curtains and muttering, *"Tick-tock, sunshine"*. I imagined the Grim Reaper pitching a tent in my garden and sharpening his scythe on the patio slabs like he'd moved in permanently.

In my mildly agitated state, I grabbed a notebook and unleashed a caffeine-fuelled tornado of ambition. Ideas poured out of me like I'd mainlined Red Bull. By breakfast, the list included juggling chainsaws on a unicycle, touring Australia as a didgeridoo-playing mime

5

artist, and bungee jumping naked over Niagara Falls.

It was chaotic. It was cathartic. It was therapeutic.

Eventually, though, even my Red Bull-fuelled optimism had to sober up. Each time I revisited the list, I trimmed a little madness. Some entries got the axe – often with a muttered, *"What the hell was I thinking?"* What remained became less adrenaline junkie and more *mortality with meaning*. My list was beginning to evolve.

Regardless of the squiggly lines above and below, one item never wavered:

Write a book.

Why, in the name of all things sensible, would anyone write a book when time itself becomes more precious than a winning lottery ticket? Honestly, I don't think I can explain it with logic. But I'll try.

The Real Book

The idea of writing wasn't a spur-of-the-moment brain burp like "go zorbing" or "underwater synchronised basket weaving." No – this one had been festering away quietly in the background for over twenty-five years. Even back then, it took another decade before I finally sat down, sharpened a pencil (optimistically, I might add), and gave it a shot.

The result? Three hundred pages of spectacular drivel. A political thriller, no less – ironic, considering my only qualification in politics is yelling at the telly during Question Time and once voting for the Monster Raving Loony Party by accident.

Somewhere around chapter twenty-three, the plot stalled like a three-legged tortoise crawling through treacle. I had no idea how to finish it (plot twist: there *was* no plot). Eventually, it was consigned to a cardboard box and carried to the shed, where it now gathers dust between a broken leaf blower and a box of old VHS tapes I've never had the heart to throw away.

My first attempt at literary greatness was a disaster of epic proportions. But the idea refused to die. It followed me around like a clingy puppy with a bladder control problem. So, when I started building my bucket list, it made the cut.

Still, I didn't exactly leap to my keyboard. Instead, I spent a ridiculous amount of time imagining what this "real" book might look like. During quiet moments – on trains, in cafés, or staring blankly out the window like a pensioner spying on neighbours – I'd daydream about dramatic scenes for a fictional narrative. Those moments brought her to life.

Cat Navarre.

My high-octane, ass-kicking heroine. A woman so impossibly gorgeous and athletic she could escape gun-toting drug cartels in South America in the morning, dismantle a bomb in Jakarta in the afternoon, and still have time before dinner to smoulder over a martini. She drove supercars like she had stolen them (because she had), dodged bullets, flirted with danger, and looked devastatingly hot while doing it.

There was only one teensy weensy snag:

I had no bloody plot.

While Cat was busy saving the world, the universe was practically dancing on my coffee table holding up neon signs which screamed, *WRITE WHAT YOU KNOW!* Did I take any notice? Of course not. I was about as observant as a goldfish in a philosophy lecture.

Then–**bam**. A digital lightning bolt struck. Two very dear friends, separately, but around the same time, reappeared in my life like the Ghosts of Sanity Past, via Facebook. Kerry H – I hadn't spoken to in over ten years. Nikki T? More like thirty. Apparently, I'm as good at keeping in touch as I am at finishing novels.

They were two of the most beautiful souls I've ever known, and somehow I'd let life carry me so far off course that I'd lost them. Probably because I was too busy being a selfish idiot.

8

We reconnected over emails and messaging apps, like a virtual reunion without the awkward buffet and "Oh God, what was your name again?" small talk.

At first, I didn't mention my diagnosis – or my bucket list. But I sent each of them an email of epic proportions. Think *War and Peace*, but with more personal anecdotes and grammatical crimes.

They both replied, with somewhat shorter emails I might add, and somewhere amid the life updates, each casually suggested I should write a book.

Now, whether that was a polite nudge or a gentle dig at my novel length email, I don't know. But their cheeky encouragement lit the fire I'd been waiting for. I had been writing to them about my life. **My real life.** And right there was the answer.

The Shift

Hindsight came rushing in like a flood through a burst dam. All those signs I'd missed. All those hours dreaming about a fictional femme fatale. And yet, there it was: I had cancer and apparently, some people thought I was handling it in an *inspirational* way.

I didn't get that, to be honest. Inspirational? Me? I was just muddling through like anyone else, only with more medical appointments and a growing appreciation for soft seating in waiting rooms.

But maybe – *just maybe* – my messy, confused, humorous, determined approach to facing terminal illness was something worth sharing. Maybe it wasn't Cat Navarre's story the world needed. Maybe it was mine.

So I finally did it. I sat down, opened a blank document, and started to write. Not about political intrigue or jungle explosions. Not about beauty, guns, and glamorous espionage. But about *me*.

Thank you, Nikki and Kerry. I love you both. xx

(And I promise to keep future emails under 10,000 words.)

Why This Book Really Exists

At first, writing this book was selfish. I just wanted to finally finish one. Like solving a Rubik's Cube or figuring out how to fold a fitted sheet properly. But when I finally told Nikki, Kerry, and later Louise G – who lost her mum to cancer – something changed.

Their encouragement shifted everything.

This book wasn't just another tick on a list. It became something else – something bigger. Maybe it could help someone else. Someone newly diagnosed. Someone who feels just as overwhelmed and unmoored as I did when I first heard the words, *incurable cancer*.

Let me be clear: I don't have the answers. I wouldn't dare claim to. I'm as qualified to dispense life advice as a chocolate teapot is to hold boiling water.

But maybe, just maybe, these pages can offer a little comfort. A little hope. A little human connection.

Maybe someone will read this and realise they're not alone.

And if that someone is you – I want you to promise me a few things

The Promises

If you're the person this book might help, right now you might feel like you're trying to climb Everest barefoot, and I know, making promises will be hard. Especially if you, like me, treat promises like sacred contracts and haven't broken one since accidentally promising my mother that I would clean my room in 1977.

But hear me out.

Promise me you'll read this book to the very end, even if I occasionally ramble like a tour guide with no map. There's a purpose behind the detours – I promise. (Though whether that purpose always makes sense is up for debate.)

Promise me you won't wave a white flag at your diagnosis. Save white flags for actual surrenders, like admitting you can't assemble IKEA furniture without crying or that you *did* in fact eat the last biscuit.

Promise me you'll love wherever and whenever you can find it. Love hard, even if it's messy, inconvenient, or covered in dog hair.

Promise me you'll laugh – even when it feels impossible. Especially when it feels impossible.

And above all...

Promise me you won't give up on living.

Not merely existing – paying bills, walking the dog,

waiting for appointments – but living. The full-contact, bruised-knees, ridiculous-mistakes, breathless-laughter kind of living.

You may have been diagnosed with a terminal illness. But you're not dead yet.

So live while you're alive.

There'll be plenty of time for sleeping when you *are* dead.

Before We Go Any Further

Let's get something out of the way before we dive into the utter chaos which is my life. Obviously, I'm not a proper writer.

With all the enthusiasm in the world, I know I'm never going to be the next J.K. Rowling. I have as much idea how these things work as a penguin has about flying a commercial aircraft.

By that logic, this book may seem a touch... disjointed. Think of it as a narrative Jenga tower: wobbly, unpredictable, and likely to collapse if you ask too many structural questions. But I promise I'll do everything I can to keep you entertained all the way to the last page – even if I have to bribe you with bad jokes, questionable metaphors, and the occasional plea to just *please* keep reading.

The next chapter starts on day one of my life and goes through to the moment in the Oncologist's suite mentioned earlier. I've tried to keep it brief, but summarising a life is like trying to fit an elephant into a matchbox: ambitious, awkward, and liable to explode.

There have been many moments which shaped me into the man writing this now – just as I'm sure there have been in your life. Hopefully yours involved fewer bad life-decisions and less tragic fashion choices in the 1980s.

What I'm about to share may seem self-indulgent. Okay, fine – it *is* self-indulgent. Like posting vacation photos online but in book form. If you only care about how I handled cancer and couldn't care less about my life's greatest hits and spectacular misses, you're welcome to skip ahead. I won't be offended. Well... maybe a little. But I'll get over it – with the help of chocolate and denial.

If, however, you choose to wade into this biographical swamp, I salute you. What you're about to read isn't fiction. It's real. The pure and unadulterated truth. Warts and all. And to save you the trouble of working it out yourself – I admit it now: I was an arrogant prick for a good portion of it.

Charlie – who you'll meet soon, and who still somehow talks to me – read the first draft and offered one of my favourite pieces of feedback ever:

"You don't come across very well." Translation: Still an arrogant prick – but at least self-aware.

She wasn't wrong. I know who I've been, and I'm not trying to sugarcoat it. I'm not looking for sympathy or validation. This story isn't about crafting a likeable protagonist, and definitely not a charm offensive. It's about telling the truth. It's about looking back at who I was, who I am, and who I might still have the time to become.

I'm not gunning for a popularity prize. (Though, if they're handing them out, I'd turn up in a tux, act surprised and graciously accept). I'm writing it for the reasons I've already laid out – reasons which hopefully made more sense a few pages ago than they do now.

So buckle up. Adjust your seat to the upright position.

We're heading into the scenic route of one man's

spectacularly imperfect life – complete with wrong turns, questionable pit stops, and the occasional breakdown on the side of the road.

Let's roll.

Jim Legging It

Just over sixty-five years ago, on a bleak and blustery Saturday night in the sweaty armpit of a British winter (think Narnia, but with more drizzle, fewer fauns, and absolutely zero chance of Turkish Delight), Jim Partington blasted out the front door of number 10, Whiteland Avenue, Bolton. He didn't so much *leave* the house as *detonate* from it in sheer panic, with no regard for dignity, warmth, or footwear.

There was no time for a scarf (a cardinal sin in the North of England), gloves, or even a final glance back at the coal fire and the armchair which still held the imprint of his backside. He simply grabbed his coat and yesterday's ill-conceived impulse buy – a teddy bear, because impending fatherhood apparently activates some primal urge to stockpile fluff – and vaulted over the doorstep like a hyperactive greyhound.

In his heroic launch, he very nearly flattened the breathless child who, moments earlier, had pounded on the door and handed him a note. A handwritten one, no less.

The note was brief. And ominous.

"It is time."

That was it. No explanation. No emojis. Just three scribbled words which sounded like a prophecy and felt like a heart attack.

The kid hadn't written it, of course. He was merely the chosen one – a pint-sized Hermes in short trousers, minus the winged sandals and with considerably more phlegm.

The year was 1959, when neighbours actually *knew* each other – *and* their business – without the need for passive-aggressive Facebook groups or anonymously posted notes about dog mess and inappropriate recycling practices. Everyone was Mr or Mrs until formally invited to drop the honourifics, and local gossip travelled faster than measles in a school canteen, thanks largely to an army of underage, underpaid couriers.

Phones did exist, but they were wall-mounted relics usually owned by the wealthier families – the ones with inside toilets and relatives who wore ties to dinner. The rest of the neighbourhood relied on what we might generously call the Emergency Child Dispatch Network.

In times of crisis or drama (births, deaths, unexpected Bake-Oven fires), the lucky few with a phone would become human switchboards. They'd answer their clunky rotary receiver, scribble notes with a stub of pencil on the back of a milk bill, then either shout vital information across the street or dispatch a local child, barefoot and bleary-eyed, like a slightly damp carrier pigeon with homework.

That night, one such child had been rudely evicted from his dreams, handed a note of ominous minimalism, and told to run like the devil himself was on roller skates behind him. And, bless his soggy little cotton socks, that's exactly what he did.

Jim, fully committed to his role as the panicking father-to-be, vanished into the inky northern night without so much as a backup plan. Through darkened parks, along icy roads, and across at least one suspiciously muddy field (shortcut? misjudged allotment? History remains unclear), he sprinted with the conviction of a man fleeing both his responsibilities *and* frostbite.

His lungs wheezed like a dying accordion, the teddy bear flailed wildly behind him like a furry distress signal, and his shoes – unsuitable for speed or dignity – slapped the pavement in rhythmic protest. He didn't own a car, of course. And had the note arrived earlier, he might've caught the last bus. But no – Bolton's mighty double-decker fleet was already tucked up back at the depot dreaming of pensioners with exact change.

Jim took the only option left open to him. He legged it.

Now, January in northern England isn't so much a month as it is an endurance test. We're talking black ice slicker than a politician's apology, breath which crystallises mid-air, and temperatures that could kill a polar bear in thermals. And yet, somehow, Jim remained upright – sweating, gasping, and regretting every life choice he'd made which didn't involve owning a motorbike or marrying someone with a car.

Eventually, he burst through the front doors of Heaton Maternity Hospital like a man arriving at the wrong audition – still clutching the teddy bear, looking like he'd run the London Marathon backwards, uphill, and in slippers.

Back in the 1950s and 60s, the very idea of fathers being allowed *anywhere near* the business end of childbirth was about as likely as finding Wi-Fi in a coal mine. It simply wasn't done. Labour was considered **a strictly female domain** – like crochet, emotional repression, and coping silently with trauma.

So Jim, a man of his era and clearly not one to break social taboos (except maybe running full-pelt through municipal shrubbery with a teddy bear), did what all respectable men did when faced with impending fatherhood: **he waited**.

Outside the maternity ward. Clutching that bear like it was both a gift and a holy relic. Trying not to pass out, throw up, or cry in front of a nurse. He sat. He stood. He paced. He made polite conversation with a vending machine. He probably questioned every decision which had led him to this moment, from the first date with my mother to the suspicious curry they'd eaten earlier that week.

Meanwhile, on the other side of those imposing doors, all hell had broken loose.

Picture this: a blazing theatre light overhead, a crack squad of midwives dressed like extras from a dystopian sci-fi film, and my poor mother – soon to be known in family lore as *My Old Dear* – mid-battle warring with the violent forces of biology. Legs up, voice at full volume, doing a pitch-perfect impression of a banshee being exorcised.

And I? I was having absolutely **none of it.**

Rather than enter the world gracefully, I decided to arrive with all the subtlety of a drunk rhino on a bouncy castle. There were limbs. There was screaming. There may have been swearing in three languages. Even the staff were beginning to look concerned.

Now, here's the thing about umbilical cords. You'd think, after nine months of faithful service keeping a foetus fed and oxygenated, they'd bow out with dignity and let the baby finish strong. **Mine had other plans.**

Apparently unwilling to go quietly, the cord decided to get a bit *hands-on* with my neck, wrapping itself around it like a boa constrictor who'd recently taken up neonatal murder as a hobby. So, the very lifeline which had kept me nourished and safe was now **actively trying to strangle me.** Classic betrayal.

My mother, to her horror, could do absolutely nothing but watch as the nurses – well-meaning but increasingly panicked – played what can only be described as a medically-themed game of "Pass the Parcel," much like it would be conducted at a five-year-olds birthday party. Only in this case, the parcel was rapidly purpling, and the music was replaced with screaming. Mostly hers.

No one seemed keen to be the one to *actually do something,* so I was tossed from one pair of hesitant arms to another like a hot potato, or maybe a radioactive ferret – nobody wanted to hold on too long.

Finally, a doctor – clearly fed up with the performance art unfolding around him – stepped in with the exasperation of a man who just wanted his tea break. I like to imagine him muttering something like, *"For heaven's sake, just unwrap the damn baby,"* before tackling me like a poorly gift-wrapped Christmas present.

After a bit of strategic unfettering and a gentle *yank*, I was freed from the cord's vice-like grip. My circulation slowly resumed, my skin returned to a colour not found in most mortuaries, and I was greeted with my first ever human interaction: **a sharp smack to the bottom.**

Ah, the warm welcome of the National Health Service. Cheers, Doc.

I responded the only way any British baby would: by crying in outrage. Loudly. Immediately. Repeatedly. I had arrived – and I had *a voice*.

With the drama momentarily subdued and the colour returning to my limbs, I was unceremoniously lobbed into what they charmingly called an **"air-tent"** – essentially a see-through box with a whiff of Victorian baby jail about it. Apparently, I needed "observation," which is medical speak for "we're not entirely sure this one's going to survive."

That slap, by the way, was the first of many disciplinary actions I'd go on to earn in life. But at least that one came with medical justification. Most others involved sarcasm and school reports.

Several days later – once the staff were satisfied that I'd stopped trying to perish dramatically – my mother and I were deemed healthy enough to leave. Or possibly just too much trouble to keep.

Dad arrived to collect us in a borrowed car, which I imagine was a rusted Morris Minor smelling faintly of petrol and boiled sweets. He had combed his hair and put on his best jumper, the one with only one suspicious stain, and was doing his best to look like he wasn't still traumatised by the midnight sprint or the fact that no one had offered him a cup of tea during the entire ordeal.

Surrounded by the hospital staff, who had witnessed my dramatic arrival and near-disastrous departure, we were escorted to the hospital exit. As we passed through the long, badly-lit corridors my shell-shocked parents were given after care tips and cheerful reassurances that, despite my brief flirtation with oxygen deprivation, I hadn't sustained any permanent damage. Physically, at least.

Mentally? Well, that was more of a grey area. My father – never one to miss an opportunity for sarcasm – would spend the next few decades blaming that fleeting lack of air for everything from my inability to sit still to my curious knack for generating absolute bedlam wherever I went.

But in those first few days, before I began my lifelong career as an agent of mild domestic anarchy, the freshly expanded Partington family enjoyed a fleeting moment of serenity. My parents basked in new-baby bliss. I slept, farted, and looked angelic. And everyone pretended that I was going to be normal.

Home Sweet Home

The first stop after my dramatic hospital debut was none other than 10 Whiteland Avenue – the very address my old man had sprinted away from like he was dodging a bookie he owed money to the night I was born. This wasn't some grand ancestral estate with sweeping driveways, ghosts in the cellar, and oil portraits cluttering the walls of a vast hallway. It was a humble three-bedroomed house tucked away in Deane, a gritty little suburb on the west side of Bolton. It belonged to my maternal grandparents – or more accurately, it was rented from the council, but let's not split hairs.

This modest semi-detached had already weathered the chaos of raising my mum and her seven siblings. It wore its emotional wallpaper and structural bruises with a certain grim pride. By the time I showed up, the eldest brother and three of Mum's sisters had flown the nest, presumably to quieter pastures where the queue for the bathroom wasn't a daily cage fight.

Two of her sisters, heartbreakingly, hadn't made it past childhood – victims of abstruse illnesses which lurked behind every doorknob before vaccines and pasteurisation became everyday miracles. No one spoke about them much, but their absence was folded into the wallpaper like an old family secret. Maybe their loss made my arrival more precious – or just more terrifying.

Still at home was Mum's younger brother, Brian, who was either thrilled or appalled to discover a squawking infant had joined the household. Even so, the house wasn't nearly as crowded as in its heyday, when the walls must have sighed with relief every time someone moved out.

For the next six months, I enjoyed the full VIP treatment. As the smallest resident and novelty attraction, I was showered with attention – chin tickles, cuddles on demand, and a chorus of *"Ooh, isn't he lovely?"* trailing me from room to room like a squeaky soundtrack. I repaid their devotion in the traditional newborn currency: erratic wailing, spectacular bowel movements, and a tireless commitment to robbing everyone of sleep like a burglar alarm no one could disarm.

Just as the household teetered on the brink of a collective breakdown, my parents scraped together enough for a deposit on a place of their own. Whether motivated by love or sheer exhaustion, who's to say – but the Partington circus packed up and rolled on.

11 Morar Drive

Our shiny new family HQ was a two-bedroom bungalow. 11 Morar Drive. It was perched on a just-built estate in Breightmet, out on Bolton's east side. To toddler me, it was nothing short of Eden: brick walls, a patch of grass, and a sandpit all of my own. Life was as easy as pie and twice as sticky. My sole daily mission was simple – squeeze every daylight hour from the street before someone forcibly hosed me down in the bath.

By the age of two or three, I'd claimed the cul-de-sac as my personal kingdom – knees permanently scabbed, nose forever running, surrounded by a gang of equally feral local kids. Back then, unleashing toddlers onto the street wasn't child endangerment; it was parenting. We flourished in an era when the gravest threat to our wellbeing was a grazed elbow, not a stranger with a van or the abyss of YouTube. In those halcyon days, the only concern was whether you'd make it home for tea – not whether you'd make it home at all.

Our gang roamed the neighbourhood like a pack of pint-sized wolves with questionable hygiene and a talent for ear-splitting shrieks. The unwritten rule was simple: if one kid showed up outdoors, the whole tribe materialised within minutes – drawn together by some magnetic toddler voodoo which baffled every adult within earshot.

The racket we generated was legendary – not mere hullabaloo but a sonic masterpiece which ricocheted through the estate. It was music to grown-up ears because it meant we were alive, accounted for, and (mostly) not setting anything on fire.

Silence, however, struck terror deep into every parent's heart. The nanosecond our clamour stopped, curtains twitched and doors flung open faster than you could mutter, *"Bloody hell, what've they done now?"* It was an instant, neighbourhood-wide fire drill – minus the fire trucks.

Fast forward to today, and street play requires high-vis vests, adult supervision, and possibly a lawyer on retainer. But in the late fifties and early sixties? Pfft. Supervision was for wimps. Traffic was laughably scarce because cars were exotic creatures most families dreamed of but couldn't afford. If a household did own one, it was about as fast as a heavily sedated sloth. Zero to sixty was more a prayer than a promise. By the time an old Morris Oxford wheezed to top speed, we'd graduated school and moved out.

On the rare occasion an ancient banger dared invade our asphalt kingdom, we executed a well-rehearsed scatter formation – a shrieking retreat to the pavement which made us look like we'd been tasered en masse. We'd applaud the driver with the fervour of royal watchers at a passing motorcade. Sometimes they'd wave back, which only fuelled our hysteria.

We were street urchins and street performers rolled into one scruffy spectacle.

Those pavement days are etched in my memory like graffiti on a school desk – some parts sweet, some stinging a little. One incident stands out brighter than a neon sign in a blackout: my first brush with canine-powered disaster.

Three doors down lived a German Shepherd – an apex predator in toddler terms – owned by one of two overgrown brothers who still lived with their Mum and Dad, giving off a whiff of permanent adolescence. The dog owner fancied himself as Bolton's answer to James Dean: black leather biker jacket, brooding air, minus any actual motorbike. I never saw him straddle anything more thrilling than a pushbike. But hey, it was the sixties – questionable fashion choices were practically mandatory.

One fine day, this furry, unleashed, battering ram clocked me from twenty yards and apparently thought, *Ah, a snack!* Next thing I knew, a slobbering missile the size of a Clydesdale horse was bearing down on my pint-sized frame. I froze like a rabbit in headlights – if the headlights were attached to a galloping hound.

In a heartbeat, I was on the pavement. One gentle nudge from that wet nose and down I went. I hit the concrete so hard I practically bounced. The human attached to the dog – our local Marlon Brando tribute act – barked orders for his canine wrecking ball to retreat. The dog obeyed with military precision. Meanwhile, I was sprawled on the ground, bawling my eyes out, convinced I'd been mauled by the Hound of the Baskervilles.

Did Biker Brother rush to check on the wailing toddler his beast had steamrolled? Of course not. He, and his dog, sauntered inside, leash dangling, gate swinging shut behind him, radiating the concern of a man who'd just spotted an interesting cloud formation.

Eventually, my sobs subsided, my dignity partially reassembled, and I resumed my adventures – a little bruised, but mostly indignant. That, dear reader, was the inaugural entry in what would become a lifelong catalogue of pratfalls, collisions, and bodily mishaps.

To this day, I wonder if that unexpected head-meets-concrete event was the grand opening act for my lifelong tinnitus – that delightful background chorus of ringing and whistling which serenades me day and night like a personal, endlessly looping elevator jingle.

Of course, the ringing isn't really in my ears at all, but in my brain – which feels like an especially mean cosmic prank from whichever department of evolution thought that was funny. Some people's tinnitus pops in and out like a nosy neighbour. Mine moved in permanently, never pays rent, and hums the same dreadful tune twenty-four-seven.

Maybe my brain just locked away the precise details of that early pavement face-plant in some vault labelled *Too Much for a Toddler, Try Again at 50*.

And you know what? Fair enough. Some things are better filed under *Best Left Vague*. Especially if it means the rest of the memories shine all the brighter.

Another memory I've retained with the kind of unnaturally vivid clarity usually reserved for humiliating moments and unpaid debts, is the day I mastered the art of riding a two-wheeled bicycle – only to have triumph violently dethroned by the gods of gravity and poor parental wardrobe choices. What started as pure elation promptly nose-dived into blood, howling, and a bit of back-alley surgery performed at the kitchen sink.

There I was, resplendent in a green, turtle-neck, woollen sweater and *beige shorts* – because apparently someone thought beige was a sensible colour for a child about to fling himself repeatedly onto the asphalt. I was pedalling furiously up and down our slightly inclined cul-de-sac like a miniature Tour de France contender with a lot more enthusiasm than skill.

The magnificent chariot I sat astride had been handed down to me by Gill, my older cousin, who had presumably outgrown both the bike and the inclination to risk life and limb atop it. And, as every child knows, when you are handed something new (or slightly second-hand but new *to you*), it absolutely must be played with immediately, without so much as a nod to common sense, safety, or the desperate pleas of concerned parents.

My Old Man was trotting alongside me, one hand gripping the back of the saddle, acting as a sort of human training wheel and insurance policy against my own lack of balance. Up and down the street we went, father and son in perfect synchrony – a partnership so noble it could have reduced Olympic coaches to tears of envy. And me? I was loving every breathless second of it.

The wind whipped against my cheeks at what I was certain must be a blistering one hundred miles per hour – though in reality, I was probably moving at the approximate pace of tectonic drift.

Then came *the moment* – that intoxicating, heart-in-throat instant when I realised Dad was no longer at my side. I turned to shout my triumph at him, only to find him standing with his arms folded, on the pavement, grinning that proud, goofy grin fathers save for their child's first monumental steps towards independence... and disaster.

I was free. Balanced. Unstoppable. A tiny master of physics and momentum. No steadying hands, no training wheels, just pure, wobbly freedom.

And then – inevitably – physics handed out a reminder as to who was the boss. In a spectacular twist of fate, my sense of balance abandoned ship faster than rats on the Titanic. One moment I was the pint-sized king of the cul-de-sac; the next, I was intimately reacquainting my knees with the pavement.

In a blur of pain and shrieking, I found myself wrapped up in the metal frame of my bike, entangled more securely than I'd ever been in my own umbilical cord – and that was a pretty impressive entanglement, according to family lore.

Cue the emergency services – a.k.a. Mum and Dad – sprinting over as though their firstborn had just survived a minor plane crash. I was extricated from the wreckage and hauled into our makeshift A&E: the draining board of the kitchen sink. There, my freshly grated knees were introduced to warm water and the liquid embodiment of Satan itself – antiseptic.

Once my shoes and socks were peeled off (taking some skin with them for good measure), Mum, armed with an industrial-size bottle of Dettol, proceeded to baptise my shredded limbs like a battlefield medic with a personal vendetta. Did the sadistic pig realise each dab felt like being stabbed with a thousand flaming needles? I howled like a werewolf under a full moon, but she pressed on relentlessly, convinced that if a little antiseptic was good, then a gallon must be positively divine. Hadn't the fall been punishment enough? Mercifully, my long-sleeved pullover spared my arms from resembling a Jackson Pollock original. Small mercies.

Now, here's the crucial takeaway, and I cannot stress this enough: if you are a parent, grandparent, or any hapless guardian entrusted with teaching a small child to ride a pushbike – DO NOT, under any circumstances, dress that child in shorts for this momentous trial.

And for the love of all things washable, never, ever choose *beige*. Beige displays everything: blood, dirt, grass stains, tears, and the undeniable evidence of catastrophic childhood incompetence. It's basically a giant billboard advertising your offspring's misadventures to the entire neighbourhood. Do your laundry (and your kid's dignity) a favour: pick dark colours.

And if you insist on ignoring this timeless wisdom – at least make sure your kitchen sink is properly sterilised. You'll need it.

Major life events continued to gate-crash my existence like uninvited relatives at a free buffet. One in particular left me ever so slightly traumatised – if not deeply suspicious of parcels wrapped in blankets: the abrupt and shady arrival of my sister, Christine.

One minute I was the undisputed golden child, basking solo in the undiluted worship of two doting parents, the centre of their domestic universe. The next minute – WHAM! There's Mum, plonked in the middle of the lounge, cradling a squishy, squeaky intruder swaddled in what looked suspiciously like *my* embroidered hospital shawl.

Where the actual fuck did that come from?

Any grown-up biological explanation to that perfectly reasonable line of enquiry would have left me more confused than a vegan judging a hog roast competition. So, in the spirit of family sanity, the finer points of human procreation were politely edited out of the official briefing.

Apparently, I'd been oblivious to the suspicious extra pounds my Old Dear had been packing beforehand – probably assuming she'd just taken a shine to pies and extra helpings of trifle. And even if I had clocked her expanding midsection, my two-year-old brain – which at the time was mostly occupied with my stuffed donkey and resisting bedtime – wouldn't have pieced it together and thought, *Ah yes, a sibling is imminent.*

So when the moment came to unveil the catastrophic breach of my personal empire, my parents chose the simplest route: plonk the new human right in front of me. Voilà – here's the living, breathing result of one too many gin-and-tonics on a drunken Saturday night nine months before.

The logic behind producing another child when the first was already more than enough trouble still baffles me. Why double the chaos? But despite the obvious signs of doom, I was weirdly thrilled. I galloped about, broadcasting to anyone with ears – and several who couldn't care less – that I now owned a *baby blister.*

Yes. Blister. Not sister. Blister. An accidental branding which, shockingly, never stuck – probably because it made her sound like something you'd pop with a sterilised needle rather than a cherished sibling.

The next nickname, though, did stick. A few years later, I started calling her *Our Kid,* and to this day it remains her official title in my head, on my tongue, and probably scribbled on a few embarrassing birthday cards.

I've never actually asked if she's okay with this permanent label – but she's never complained, so I assume she's either perfectly fine with it or quietly stockpiling decades of sibling payback while I remain blissfully unaware. Either way, the golden child survived the coup. Just about.

Academia

At the scandalously mature age of four, I embarked on my grand academic odyssey at Crompton Fold Primary School – a place so mythical in my mind that most of my memories of it could fit on a postage stamp, and still leave room for the King's head.

Ask me what I learned there? I've got nothing. But I do remember Duncan – the only classmate whose face didn't vanish into the misty fog of pre-school amnesia. Duncan was my first best mate and our friendship was forged in the fires of matching green turtle-neck sweaters – the kind of crime against fabric which would get your parents jailed for child endangerment today. Nothing bonds small children quite like being equally humiliated by your guardians' sense of 'fashion'.

Duncan and I were inseparable for approximately five minutes, which in four-year-old terms is equivalent to a lifelong brotherhood. Naturally, destiny would cruelly rip us apart before we could even swap snack boxes properly – but more on that shortly.

Now, if you're hoping for some riveting tales from inside the classroom, prepare yourself for crushing disappointment. My goldfish-level attention span meant I absorbed about as much knowledge as a brick absorbs rainwater. But what I *do* remember – in glorious technicolour and Dolby Surround Sound – is the daily trek to and from that hallowed institution.

Modern children are chauffeured about in climate-controlled SUVs with Bluetooth playlists and heated cup holders. I had sturdy shoes and a mother with laser vision, deployed behind our living-room curtains. She'd peek out like a Cold War spy to ensure her beloved offspring didn't spontaneously combust before reaching the corner of our street.

At that corner, I met up with Gill – my cousin, mentor, and reluctant babysitter – who doubled as the original 'designated driver' of our pedestrian convoy. She lived down at the far end of Morar Drive and was also the charitable soul who handed down to me the pre-loved pushbike which had already tried to kill me.

Gill's job was clear: keep me alive long enough to learn the alphabet. My mother's standing instruction to me was gospel: *"Whatever Gill says, you do – or so help me God, there will be consequences which will make the Spanish Inquisition look like a pillow fight."* Not that rebellion crossed my mind. Gill was my personal hero – half angel, half commando – and I would have followed her to Mordor if she'd asked.

Our school route wound through shadowy back alleys and along roaring main roads – the sort of adventure which would trigger twelve local Facebook groups and a full-scale search party nowadays. But Gill, at the ancient and wise age of seven, patrolled our path with the vigilance of a Royal Bodyguard, yanking me out of the path of oncoming traffic and denying me the thrill of leaping into every muddy puddle we passed.

I obeyed because Gill was everything. Even as a snot-nosed tot, I knew she was cool. She had a room. She had secrets. She had *records*.

Years later, she dragged me into her sacred teenage cave with the urgency of someone about to reveal the cure for boredom itself. *"You have to hear this,"* she declared, wide-eyed, as if she'd discovered rock and roll's version of the Holy Grail.

Obedience was hardwired into my DNA by this point, so I perched on her bed, bracing myself for... who knows? Maybe a lecture on why boys shouldn't eat worms? But instead, Gill flipped open her glorious red record player with the solemn grace of Indiana Jones lifting a golden idol.

Out came the black vinyl disc – a forty-five which might as well have been forged in the fires of Mount Doom. She dropped the stylus into the groove, and for a few seconds, there was that heavenly crackle, that whisper of anticipation – and then...

OMG!

A distorted guitar riff exploded out of nowhere, rattling the windows and rearranging my internal organs. It was raw, it was loud, it was everything polite society warned you about. My feet betrayed me immediately, twitching and tapping like I'd been zapped with a cattle prod. Then a voice – a voice so cool, so dripping with swagger it practically oozed glitter – took over my brain.

Before I knew it, I was airborne. Downstairs, my poor parents, Aunties and Uncles , probably thought the ceiling was about to cave in as their beloved son went full Tasmanian Devil in Gill's bedroom. I was spinning, flailing, inventing new dance moves which looked suspiciously like medical emergencies.

Fun fact: I couldn't dance then. I can't dance now. But Marc Bolan and T.Rex didn't care – they wanted you moving, even if it meant your limbs threatened innocent bystanders. That single moment cracked open my world like a Fabergé egg. I didn't just *hear* rock and roll; it possessed me, rewiring my soul in sequins and swagger.

Right – back to four-year-old me, strutting around like a big shot with exactly three months of 'education' under my belt. My morning ritual was the tightest operation in town. At precisely eight o'clock, Mum would appear beside my bed, applying just enough shoulder tap to resurrect my consciousness from the dead. This was no mere shake – this was a spiritual extraction, coaxing my drooling spirit back from whatever monster-infested dreamscape I'd been exploring.

Next, Mum transformed into the world's least magical fairy – housecoat, curlers, the whole glamorous ensemble – and flung open the world's most ineffective curtains. Blinding daylight punched me straight in the retinas, and with it, my fragile hope of more sleep evaporated. My bed, my beloved fortress of warmth and snotty dreams, became no safer than an inflatable dinghy in a shark tank.

Meanwhile, across the room, my baby sister, Christine, lay perfectly still on her back, eyes unblinking, staring at the ceiling as if decoding alien Morse code. She never cried. She never threw up on visiting relatives. She just *watched*. Even at four, I suspected she wasn't so much a baby as an undercover alien life form gathering intel on our species.

After the ceremonial waking came the dressing ritual

– a seamless collaboration between my half-asleep limbs and Mum's saintly patience. I was expected to insert arms and legs into the appropriate holes while Mum managed the engineering marvel of buttons, zips, and shoe laces, muttering ancient motherly incantations under her breath.

Thus armed in my school uniform, I was dispatched to the kitchen to ingest cereal while Mum checked on our resident extraterrestrial.

And then, one day...

Well, let's just say the universe decided to flip the table.

The Road To Somewhere

I was woken in the usual gentle way every school morning: a motherly whisper, a gentle tap or two on my shoulder, and a faint hope that I might open my eyes without a fight. But this morning, something smelled fishier than a seaside chip shop. The flimsy curtains – those threadbare bits of cloth which wouldn't keep out a searchlight, let alone daylight – stayed shut tight. And yet, it was pitch black outside. I knew this because I was an expert in pre-dawn grumpiness, and this was *well* before any decent human ought to be conscious.

Instead of my usual bleary-eyed rummage for clean socks among suspiciously crunchy ones, my clothes were laid out at the foot of my bed like a tiny shrine to mischief. But they weren't my proper, respectable school uniform which made me look like a trainee accountant. No, these were my play clothes: the battle-scarred shorts and shirt I usually wore to climb trees, fall out of them, and come home covered in grass stains and questionable bruises.

Adding to this unfolding Twilight Zone episode, the wardrobe and chest of drawers seemed to have vanished altogether. I half expected Rod Serling to step out of the shadows and narrate my fate. Instead, I heard Dad banging about in the kitchen – which meant he hadn't gone to work yet. In my four-year-old logic, this left two possible explanations: either it was the crack of doom, or Mum had finally gone round the bend.

Once dressed – with the help of a parental pat on the

bum, a time-honoured signal for "get a move on, Short Stuff" – I was dispatched to the kitchen, leaving Mum to tend to Christine, the family's resident enigma. As usual, she lay in her cot, eyes glued to the ceiling as if decoding ancient hieroglyphs only she could see. Perhaps, she was just contemplating life's great questions, like "Why do big people make such weird noises when they bend over?"

Meanwhile, I sat on the kitchen floor, chomping cereal from a plastic bowl like a half-feral puppy. Something else caught my beady, little eye: the table and chairs were missing. In fact, the lounge room looked suspiciously empty too, as if burglars had come in the night and politely removed only the bulky furniture. I glanced at Mum and Dad, hoping for a clue, but they carried on as though nothing had happened. Apparently, in the 1960s, if your house got half-pinched, you just had your Cornflakes and waited for further instructions.

Eventually, the grand secret was revealed: Mum wasn't loopy, Dad wasn't going to work, and – drumroll, please – I wasn't going to school. Nope. I was going on an *adventure* in a giant truck waiting at the end of the drive.

I bolted to the bay window and pressed my nose against the glass like a tiny undercover agent. Through the gloom, I spied our new chariot: an enormous truck, the sort which looked big enough to carry a three-ring circus, a few elephants, and possibly a moon rocket. Naturally, I had to get outside to inspect this beast immediately. There, stacked in the back, was the solution to our furniture's sudden vanishing act – everything we owned was crammed inside.

From my garden gnome vantage point on the

pavement, the truck seemed like a skyscraper on wheels, though in reality, it was probably no bigger than a Hi-top Ford Transit. But to a boy fuelled by imagination and sugar, it was practically the Starship Enterprise.

Before the sun even bothered clocking on for the day, Dad and I climbed aboard our mechanical juggernaut. With a sound which could be likened to a herd of metal goats, Dad "coaxed" the truck into gear, which required the grace of a blacksmith performing open-heart surgery. We trundled down Morar Drive for the very last time, me buzzing with excitement, Dad pretending to know what he was doing.

Bear in mind, this was the era before synchromesh gearboxes – those smooth marvels which let you change gear without waking the dead. What we had was a crash box, a medieval torture device for truck drivers' ears and egos. Every gear change was a violent duet of grinding metal and Dad muttering words I was told not to repeat in front of my Mother. But to me, each clang and crunch was another note in the glorious symphony of adventure. There was, however, one tiny detail left unexplained: where on Earth were we going, and why were we running away in the middle of the night?

The answer turned out to be St Annes-on-the-Sea, a coastal town in north-west England which snuggles under Blackpool on the map like its shy younger sibling. It was only about forty miles north-west of my native Bolton – a distance so laughable that even the local pigeons would've rolled their eyes and ordered a taxi rather than fly it.

As its name hints, St Annes is perched right where the

42

River Ribble shakes hands with the Irish Sea, probably arguing over who gets to taste saltier that day.

By the time we arrived, my internal organs felt like they'd been thoroughly re-arranged by the truck's non-existent suspension. These days, I am licensed to drive modern Australian road trains which glide along like armchairs on wheels – cup holders, air con, seats designed by actual humans. That old rental truck, however, was apparently engineered by someone who thought comfort was for sissies and seat padding was optional. It treated both our furniture *and* our spines with equal contempt.

So, what prompted this grand escape to the seaside?

One word: Mum. She had history. Just as she'd once charmed Dad into buying 11 Morar Drive in Breightmet, I suspect the bracing, smog-free sea air of St Annes had tickled her fancy during one of our regular visits to her royal relatives: Auntie Doris and Uncle Stan – who, in an impressive display of family co-dependence, lived right next door to each other.

I imagine the conversation went something like this:

Mum: "Isn't it lovely here?"

Dad: [with a trapped look in his eyes] "Yes, dear."

And that was that. Fast-forward to us barrelling down the road in a borrowed truck.

During one of these so-called "just a quick visit" trips – which were obviously covert reconnaissance missions – Mum spotted a 'For Sale' sign on a house directly opposite Stan's. Probably love at first sniff of fresh sea breeze. An offer was made and, miracle of miracles, accepted. Even though the sale was flimsier than the curtains back home, we packed up and moved anyway. Because in my family, we didn't do "waiting patiently for paperwork." We did "wing it and hope for the best."

Since the new house wasn't quite ours yet, we moved into Auntie Doris's place like well-mannered squatters. This worked out brilliantly for me because Doris had a son, Glenn, eight months older than me – which, in kid years, made him practically a wise old sage. Instantly, I had a new cousin and a new best mate rolled into one. Poor Duncan back in Bolton, with his permanently knitted green jumper, was forgotten quicker than you could say "good riddance, itchy wool." Partington life was off to a flying start for me.

Sadly, my parents' luck had the lifespan of a mayfly. No sooner had the last armchair been wedged precariously into Doris's dining room than the house seller suddenly changed their mind. Deal off. Just like that. No reason given. Probably decided they didn't want a grubby family of ceiling-gazers moving into the street.

This threw my folks into what historians might describe as a "complete bloody shambles." Our Bolton house was already sold – contracts signed, deposit spent, and Dad had accepted a new job in St Annes, due to start in a couple of months. I'd been registered at my new school, ready to inflict my charm on fresh teachers, and Christine had already located the next ceiling to stare into. There was no going back.

They might have set fire to the furniture and claimed insurance, but fate tossed them a lifeline in the form of another 'For Sale' sign – this time next door to Auntie Doris's. It cost five hundred quid more (a fortune in the 60s – roughly equivalent to a year's wages plus one healthy kidney), but Dad coughed up the extra to save his sanity and our family from becoming permanent couch-surfers.

And so, we began our new life in St Annes: slightly broker, a bit more dishevelled, but officially seaside folk at last. Christine had a fresh ceiling to interrogate, Mum had her salty air, and Dad had a new mortgage and a thousand new grey hairs. As for me? I had Glenn, the beach, and a truckload of new mischief to get into. Not a bad trade for an early wake-up call.

New Town, New Schools

And so began our new life in St Annes–complete with ceiling-staring babies and the nagging suspicion we'd just fallen victim to the most courteous real estate ambush in the history of Britain.

We rolled up on November 6th, and to this day I couldn't tell you if I started school that very week or if I was mercifully given the sweet reprieve of Christmas first. What I *do* remember – vividly – is discovering that I wouldn't be going to the same school as Glenn. Honestly, it was like finding out Father Christmas was just your dad after six pints, crammed into a moth-eaten red suit he'd borrowed from the pub's fancy-dress box.

Apparently, St Thomas's, where Glenn went, had hit its legal limit for unruly children, so they shipped me off to St Annes County Primary instead – better known to everyone as Sydney Street, because the Victorians had all the imagination of a wet dishcloth when it came to naming things.

Day one, I'm plonked down at a table with four lads: Chris K, Dave C, Barry K, and Glenn F (not my cousin, a new Glenn – Glenns were abundant back then). Sweet mother of chaos, I'd stumbled into a goldmine of pint-sized lunacy. These boys were a glorious tornado of mischief: they'd make you laugh so violently you'd snort milk out of your nose *without* having drunk any. By lunch I knew two things: one, school was about to get a lot more entertaining; and two, my teachers would age faster than a snowball in a heatwave.

Despite our daily efforts to push our educators to the brink of early retirement, I'm proud to report these menaces are now respectable adults – living proof that youthful delinquency doesn't necessarily end in prison time. Chris and I still keep the friendship alive – detentions really do forge unbreakable bonds. He moved back to St Annes after years in the States, probably spinning the Yanks tall tales about British school dinners and a casual bit of corporal punishment. He's now our unofficial class gossip hotline – if someone we know sneezes in St Annes, Chris texts me about it.

My Sydney Street adventures were mostly harmless – if you overlook the occasional caning, which back then was the go-to solution for pretty much anything short of arson. Late for assembly? WHACK. Didn't say please? WHACK. Smirked at the dinner lady? WHACK. It was like living inside a Monty Python sketch.

One particularly memorable incident, though, skipped the bamboo cane entirely. A few of us eight-year-old master criminals staged what I still maintain was a victimless crime: we liberated an entire shelf's worth of pens and notebooks from the local stationer. Think Robin Hood, only instead of stealing from the rich and giving to the poor, we stole from the stationary aisle and gave to ourselves.

Unfortunately, our criminal genius fell apart at the 'not getting caught' stage – we laid out our loot proudly on our desks the next day like a black-market jumble sale. Some nosey do-gooder grassed us up. The headmistress, clearly worried she'd snap her cane on this one, went nuclear and tattled straight to our parents. I'd have happily taken the flogging over *that* phone call.

By 1970, I was eleven, Sydney Street was almost behind me, and the Eleven Plus exam loomed like a career-ending penalty kick. Pass, and you were king of the castle at Grammar School. Fail, and it was Ansdell Secondary Modern – a place so uninspiring even your dreams had to nap there. Boys went to King Edward VII Grammar; girls to Queen Mary's. Fail, and you all ended up together at Ansdell – future rock stars and petty criminals alike.

King Teds came with a catch: no football. Instead, they offered Rugby – basically an organised excuse for bigger boys to flatten smaller boys into the mud. I was all about the beautiful game – dreaming of being George Best, Bobby Charlton, or Geoff Hurst (spoiler: I was none of these).

Part of me thought about failing on purpose–self-sabotage for the greater footballing good – but I was never bright enough to flunk convincingly. Even if I'd tried, my mother had a cunning Plan B: a private entrance exam which had I passed would ensure I'd get into King Ted's. The cost of my education would have been the equivalent of giving an arm and a leg, but Mother Dear would have secured the bragging rights at the local butchers. Thankfully, I passed and was given the free route allowing Dad's golf fund to survive another day.

Bonus: Cousin Glenn and nearly the whole gang – Chris, Dave, Barry – passed too. I wasn't going alone; I had my band of merry idiots.

Six years later, I'd mastered a mountain of knowledge I've never used since. Latin verbs? Forgotten. Pythagoras? Useless. Historical dates? Pub Trivia quiz night fodder at best. In 1975, I somehow scraped through six O-levels, convincing my mother I was destined for Oxford or Cambridge (in her head, anyway). Had her wish come true, I could imagine her dropping this fact on complete strangers in the queue for fish fillets: "Our *Andrew* – off to university, don't you know!" Despite my protests that I was called Andy, not Andrew, she persisted–possibly in case the neighbours thought she'd raised a hooligan. Maybe she had.

She convinced me to stay on at school and study A levels, the path to Uni, while my mates bagged glamorous apprenticeships at British Aerospace (working on actual planes!) or cushy computer programmer gigs at Guardian Royal Exchange. I was stuck learning Applied Maths, Physics, and Art – a trio which made as much sense together as a fish riding a bicycle, while they were earning real money.

If I'd stayed the course, I'd probably have ended up an architect with a beard, a roll of blueprints, and ready to engage in heated arguments about bricks. But the universe – and my spontaneous streak – had other plans.

Just over halfway through my first A-Level year, spring rolled in, the daffodils bloomed, and I found myself in Batman's office yet again facing serious charges. Batman, our caped headmaster – not because he fought crime and drove a bat-mobile, but because he roamed the halls in a flowing academic gown which made him look like a vampire moonlighting as a Latin teacher.

I can't remember exactly what crime I had committed that time. Could've been the shoulder-length hair, the forged sick note, or the day I told a Physics teacher – in front of the entire class – that he was a "motherf******* goat-shagger." Not exactly a career highlight for my diplomacy skills. But, whatever crime it was, the punishment, and I would be punished, was going to be heavy use of a cane. It all boiled down to a teacher's word against mine, an argument I was never going to win.

Prior to him performing his sadistic art, Batman did his usual: dramatic pacing, theatrical lecturing, a build-up allowing the "canee" to dwell much longer on the anticipation of the pain to come. Quite often the fear of punishment is worse than the punishment itself. The vicious bastard was going to eke out every ounce of pleasure from the moment.

He was mid-monologue, droning on like a broken lawnmower, when I drifted off to Andy-land (my favourite holiday spot). Sudden silence snapped me back. He was staring at me like I owed him rent.

"Do tell," he said, maybe for the second time.

I had no idea what he had just said. I panicked and blurted out the first thing which popped into my head:

"Sixth form's not for me. This is my last day."

He did not take my impromptu resignation well. He wheezed and spluttered like an asthmatic tractor, and stomped back and forth muttering about responsibility, squandered opportunity, and probably the downfall of

50

modern civilisation.

By then, I'd tuned him out again, watching this once terrifying tyrant deflate like a punctured beach ball. All the fear he'd once commanded over me was evaporating as I realised: he had no power anymore.

"We're done here," I said, and meant it.

I walked out – no plan, no regrets. Collected my stuff from my locker, waltzed out the sacred staff doors (reserved for Batman's dramatic entrances), and marched up the long school drive, shedding six years of rules like confetti at a wedding.

Through the iron gates, onto Clifton Drive – air fresher, sun brighter. I was free.

And then it hit me.

Oh. Bugger.

What the hell was I going to tell Mum and Dad?

I didn't know then, of course, but winging it would become my life's greatest skill – and sometimes, the best adventures really do begin with a door slammed behind you and absolutely no idea what comes next.

Time To Grow Up

During most of my secondary school years, I worked outside school hours – not because I was a budding workaholic, but because I was always saving for some must-have item which no amount of polite begging, strategic sulking, or subtle guilt-tripping would ever extract from my parents. They made sure I had the necessities – food, clothing, a roof over my head – but luxuries? Forget it. If I wanted something Santa Claus wasn't bringing (and his gift budget seemed about as generous as my dad's wallet on curry night), I had to fund my teenage whims myself through the ancient art of actual work. So I did.

From Monday to Saturday, I earned what could generously be described as a microscopic income by delivering fresh-off-the-printer copies of *The Blackpool Evening Gazette* to houses along a predetermined route. This job paid what my grandmother would have called "pin money" – which is to say, barely enough to buy actual pins, let alone anything worth bragging about to your mates. I was essentially a human newspaper-dispensing machine, trudging through the streets of St Annes like a very slow, weather-dependent Amazon Prime.

But the weekend – ah, the weekend was when I raked in the big bucks! Well, relatively big bucks. Big bucks by the standards of a teenager whose previous wealth had been measured in pocket fluff and lost coppers found behind the sofa.

On Saturdays and Sundays, I was up at the crack of dawn in summer and at some ungodly pre-dawn hour in winter. Even the roosters were hitting the snooze button at that time, and I envied them deeply. I'd be scooped up from the pavement outside my house by a local milk deliveryman in his battered Ford Transit. The back of the van was stacked to the roof with rattling crates of milk, which we'd distribute noisily to doorsteps throughout town, often waking up half the street with our expert bottle-clanking technique. By 10 a.m., all the full bottles were gone. All we had on board were the empties and my frozen fingers.

How about that? It was the '70s, and milk was delivered by the pint in glass bottles. We'd rock up at a doorstep with a couple of pints and find the empties from the day before waiting like loyal soldiers ready for redeployment. At the end of the round, the empties went back to the dairy, got boiled alive, refilled, and sent out again. No plastic bins, no blue bags, no angry seagulls tearing open your recycling – just old-school, squeaky-clean glass. Greta Thunberg would have wept tears of pure joy.

After the milk round, I was off to job number two, because apparently one borderline-illegal child labour gig wasn't enough for my ambitious little self.

In summer, St Annes was like Las Vegas without the lights, gambling, or fun – but with twice as many dodgy chip shops. From mid-April to late September, tourists – mostly from grim northern towns where coal dust doubled as exfoliant – flooded in to fill their lungs with bracing, clean sea air and their bellies with food which probably failed every health inspection known to man. This was pre-EasyJet, remember, when "cheap flights" were just a mad scientist's dream, and Benidorm for the weekend was about as realistic as teleportation.

The locals, bless them, welcomed these visitors like long-lost relatives – relatives who happened to spit out cash with every stick of rock they bought. Hotels scrambled to hire extra staff, transforming overnight from peaceful mausoleums to frantic anthills of bad tempers and worse pay. Chefs earned decent wages because they could cook actual food which didn't poison people. Waiters and waitresses? Paid peanuts, but cunning enough to hoover up tips from tourists who'd drowned all financial sense in three bottles of house red.

Then there was me – so far down the hotel food chain I practically lived underground. I was a Pot Washer, which sounds quite regal until you spend five minutes wrist-deep in industrial dishwater that's 10% grease, 90% regret.

The money wasn't exactly life-changing, but for a kid eyeing up a reel-to-reel tape recorder or a pair of George Best Stylo Matchmaker boots – the kind which would magically transform me from last pick on the pitch to local football deity – it was a fortune. Teenage financial cheat code unlocked!

I worked at the Bedford Hotel, which wasn't the biggest or flashiest place in town, but it kept me busier than a one-armed wallpaper hanger in a wind tunnel every weekend. During school holidays, the owner kindly exploited me for even more hours, comforted by the fact that my minimum wage didn't come with complaints. My battered old biscuit tin – my personal Fort Knox – rattled happily all summer long.

Then came The Great Exit – my spontaneous, heroic storming out of the Bat Cave (a.k.a. King Teds' headmaster's lair). I like to think he still talks about me to this day, possibly with a twitch in his left eye.

The paper round and milk gig became casualties of my newfound freedom, sacrificed on the altar of pretending to be an adult. They'd served their purpose when I had to wear a uniform and pretend to care about timetables. Now I was a free agent – an educational drop-out with a pressing need to look like I had a plan, even if my entire plan was, basically: "wing it."

Luckily, I kept the Bedford Hotel gig. Tourists were about to descend in their donkey-jacketed thousands, and my wallet needed feeding. Then my mate Chris Riley – the human Swiss Army knife of local hospitality – pulled some strings and landed me a spot at his hotel instead. Same pot washing, but more hours and a better hourly rate. I was practically a teenage tycoon.

Of course, earning money is one thing – having ambitions is another. Mum decided I should be the next Frank Lloyd Wright, mainly because I once glued some Air-fix kits together without sticking my fingers to the dog. The town was sprouting boring new buildings that looked like giant shoeboxes, and I convinced myself I could do better.

To become an architect, I'd have to crawl back to school, pass three A-Levels, and charm every teacher into forgetting I'd once called them "soulless time vampires." Applied Maths? Maybe. Physics? No problem. But Art?

Why, in the name of everything sacred, did I choose Art?

I couldn't draw a matchstick man without him looking like he'd survived multiple hip surgeries and a bar fight. Unless A-Level Art pivoted overnight to "emulsion rolling and skirting board glossing," I was done for. The syllabus wanted sweeping landscapes and fruit bowls which looked like you could nick an apple off the canvas. My style was more "decorator's mate after four pints."

Van Gogh had ear issues; I had talent issues. So architecture went the same way as my school career – filed under "Nice Idea, Next!"

Becoming an Architect was as likely as me becoming the next James Bond. But an Architectural Technician? That was achievable – like finding a £20 note in a coat you haven't worn in years.

What's an Architectural Technician, you ask? It's basically the poor sod who takes the architect's fanciful doodles and translates them into practical instructions so the builders don't mutiny halfway through. Think dream killer with a T-square. No endless university slog – just a day-release course at the local college, a measly five-year qualification stretch (about the same as waiting for a bus in winter), and a steady pay-cheque while my sanity eroded one blueprint at a time.

I wrote letters. I licked so many stamps I developed a mild adhesive dependency. Miraculously, I landed two job offers as a Trainee Architectural Technician – I was briefly a hot commodity! Naturally, I chose the one where an ex-girlfriend's father didn't work. Not because I'm petty (I absolutely am), but because the prospect of daily death stares from a man who'd once threatened to break my nose didn't appeal. Picky, I know.

Mum bragged to the neighbours like I'd just invented penicillin. *"He's in the professions now!"* she'd beam, while I lived on Pot Noodles and existential dread. In the '70s, a trainee anything meant you were paid in magic beans and forced optimism, with the faint promise of a proper wage someday – assuming you didn't spectacularly cock it up.

Obviously, I kept my hotel side hustle. Something had to pay for the beer I was rapidly developing a taste for, and to keep my beloved (read: rusting) Morris 1300 coughing along the dual carriageway sounding like a cement mixer full of metal cutlery.

Speaking of beer... sometimes we paid for it. Other times, not so much. By "we," I mean me and Chris – my partner-in-crime, moral compass (badly calibrated), and co-architect of terrible decisions.

Chris spent summers as a suave waiter but was often dragged into last-minute Night Porter shifts when Keith, the full-time porter, lost his heroic battle with sobriety. Keith's daily routine after an all night shift, involved sleeping until lunch, then propping up his favourite pub bar until he resembled an inflatable wacky waving tube man – only smellier. Come shift time, Keith would, quite often, be so marinated in ale he'd need divine intervention and a forklift to clock in.

Cue Chris, the hotel's secret backup plan. One call to tell him Keith had "Done it again!" And he hot footed it over to the hotel to stand in.

It was an easy gig as the elderly guests were all snoring by 10 p.m., leaving Chris with little to do and the bar deserted.

At precisely 11:00 p.m., the on-duty bar staff would have their work domain all spick and span and by 11:01 p.m. they were heading for home. At 11:02 p.m., I'd sneak in through the staff entrance like a low-budget burglar, creep past the kitchen, and find Chris on his knees with a screwdriver, picking the service door lock like a safecracker with zero moral compass. Once inside, we poured free pints, debated life's big questions, and single-handedly destroyed the hotel's profit margins.

Management's stock checks were about as frequent as Halley's Comet, so we went undetected until our own stupidity intervened.

One night, emboldened by at least six too many lagers, we decided to sample the expensive liqueurs and top-shelf whiskey – the bottles which practically had "Do Not Touch Unless Your Dad Owns a Yacht" written on them.

Cut to the next morning: the breakfast staff found us passed out on the sun lounge sofas, reeking of crème de menthe and Glenfiddich. Not exactly rock stars – more like bargain-bin Degenerates Anonymous.

They sacked us so fast it left a friction burn. But, bafflingly, some divine paperwork mix-up meant we were quietly re-hired a week later. Maybe they appreciated our dedication to quality control.

Chris's unofficial porter career ended, and suddenly the bar had security locks which were so sophisticated they might as well have required retinal scanners to unlock them. Even we weren't stupid, or clever enough, to challenge those. Sometimes wisdom comes disguised as humiliation and a monster hangover.

I stuck at being an architectural technician for two years – two glorious years of squinting at blueprints, wrestling tracing paper, and praying my calculations wouldn't bring entire buildings crashing down. Then a practice in St Annes offered double the pay and bigger projects – naturally, I accepted. Who wouldn't want to earn twice the money to be twice as terrified of making mistakes?

Chris, meanwhile, trumped me spectacularly by landing a gig at some swanky Geneva hotel – the sort of place where royalty and presidents argue over whose slippers are fluffier. Bond villain territory. Our petty crime spree screeched to a halt overnight.

So there we were: him in Geneva, me in St Annes. Forced into respectable adulthood for a whole year – like a prison sentence with pay stubs. With Chris gone, the lock-picking, pint-pilfering, and questionable ethics dried up. And for the first time in my life, I did what I never thought possible: I focused solely on work.

Yes, me. Focusing. Miracles happen.

At the new practice, I operated like some sort of architectural vending machine – feed me a planning application and out popped a shiny new building,

59

complete with working plumbing and doors which mostly opened the right way. Every time I finished a project, I was rewarded with a bigger, fancier contract. Capitalism at its most intoxicating.

But wait – like every bad infomercial – there's more! Two drawing services somehow heard I was basically the Picasso of planning permission (architectural gossip spreads faster than an STD in a university dorm). They offered to throw extra work my way on a job-by-job basis.

So there I was, moonlighting as a double agent: by day, a buttoned-up office drone producing respectable structures which didn't collapse (always a bonus); by night, a freelance plan-slinger knocking out kitchen extensions, roof lifts, and garage conversions I could practically draw with my eyes closed. The best part? It was all under the table – pure, untraceable cash flowing into my pockets like Niagara Falls in pound coins. I was earning more than I'd dreamed possible five years earlier – and miraculously, I hadn't cocked anything up. Yet.

Then disaster struck in the most delightfully inconvenient way imaginable: Chris came home.

Now don't get me wrong – his return wasn't the catastrophe. I was ecstatic. Truly. Seeing him again felt like stumbling across your favourite kebab shop still being open after closing time at the local.

We hit the pubs, swapped heroic tales of adulthood, and picked up exactly where we'd left off: two idiots with slightly better haircuts and marginally improved hygiene. He regaled me with stories of Geneva's high society – dignitaries, diplomats, and questionable fondue etiquette

– while I dazzled him with thrilling accounts of drawing rectangles for money. Best mates again, older and debatably wiser.

It was the run-up to Christmas and, because we were legends in our own lunch breaks, word got out faster than a pub rumour that Chris was back in town. Suddenly, invitations to every half-decent shindig poured in – we were a two-man travelling party, booked solid in the lead-up to the big day. The grand finale? A Christmas Eve knees-up in a flat conveniently located around the corner from my parents' house. Handy for both mischief and a short, shame-faced stagger home.

Chris hailed from the kind of good, church-going folk who not only knew where the local parish was but actually went there – willingly. On Christmas Eve, his entire clan gathered for a holy service near their home, joined this year by a visiting family friend staying at a hotel in Blackpool. Ever the saintly soul (and maybe angling for a halo upgrade), Chris nobly volunteered to remain stone-cold sober and play taxi driver for this guest, dropping her back at her hotel after the service.

Meanwhile, my own faithful squadron of merry lunatics had already set up base camp at a nearby pub, determined to single-handedly keep the brewing industry afloat.

Chris swung by with the family friend in tow to let me know that once his chauffeur duties were done, he'd double back to Julian's – our designated headquarters for the late-night revelry.

Now, this family friend was – and I'm not exaggerating

61

– so drop-dead gorgeous she could have caused a traffic pile-up just by stepping outside. She had the sort of looks which turned grown men into stammering puddles of idiocy. Chris didn't have to say a word – one quick flash of his signature grin said it all: if his luck held, I wouldn't be seeing him until Easter. I fired back my own grin: *Good luck, Romeo. See you when you come up for air.*

And then – the party of all parties unfolded. The stuff of legend. The kind that makes you question your life choices while also bragging about them for years afterward. Chris, unsurprisingly, never turned up – but not because he'd been lost in romantic bliss. Oh no. Quite the opposite, in fact.

Come Boxing Day, I was propped up in our regular café, looking like something the cat dragged in, rolled through a hedge, and abandoned for dead. My hangover had a hangover. I was clutching a coffee the size of a small bucket, praying it would resurrect what few brain cells I had left, when the door slammed open like a scene from a soap opera.

In stormed Jayne B, a local regular who'd known me since my biggest worry was who'd nicked my pudding at lunch. She made a beeline for me at warp speed, skipping the usual pleasantries like *hello* and *are you alive?*

"It's Chris!" she gasped, words slicing through my fuzzy brain like a chainsaw through butter. "He's in a coma at the hospital!"

And just like that, I was sober.

Christopher John Riley

I have no recollection of the drive from the Blue Fountain Coffee Lounge to Blackpool Victoria Hospital. I don't remember how I found out which ward Chris was in. All I remember is standing next to his mum in the Intensive Care Unit. She turned to me and gently said, *"Go in and see him."*

The door opened into a dimly lit room. Chris lay motionless on a hospital bed, a silver, foil-like blanket draped over him. Wires and sensors snaked across his chest. A small tube fed into his nose; a larger one hung from the side of his mouth. I don't remember what they were connected to – maybe I never looked. His chest rose and fell beneath the blanket, half-covered, as machines around him clicked and beeped softly.

Was he in a coma? Or just asleep? I had no way of knowing. All I knew was that my best mate was in that bed, unreachable.

"Talk to him. He might respond to your voice," the young nurse said as she moved around, checking monitors, adjusting tubes. Or at least, that's what I think she was doing.

I sat down beside him, staring.

What the fuck was happening to my best mate?

This wasn't just someone I knew. This was Chris – my closest friend. The person I'd laughed with, fought with, grown up with. We were never quiet around each other. Put us in a room, and it would be filled with our voices, stories, relentless banter. But now? I couldn't think of a single thing to say. I couldn't even cry. I was completely, painfully mute.

"Talk to him," the nurse repeated, a little softer this time.

Talk to him? About what?

Eventually, I began to speak. I told him about Julian's party. About who had shown up, the ridiculous dance moves, the songs we had played air-guitar to. But as the words left my mouth, guilt crept in – sharp and sudden. How could I have been having a good time while Chris was... here?

I fell silent and glanced up at the nurse, ashamed. She met my eyes and gave me a small, kind smile. A nod, as if to say, *It's okay. Keep going.*

So I did. Awkwardly at first, stumbling through memories. But like anything you do for the first time, the strangeness faded. Talking to Chris – one-sided as it was – began to feel almost normal. I was talking *with* him, not *at* him. Like I always   had.

I don't remember how long I sat there that first time, but eventually the nurse came over and gently suggested I take a break so his mum could come back in. As I stood up, she added with a faint grin, "You two really know how to party."

I must've said something about our antics. I don't recall what exactly, but for her to say that – I must've brought him to life for a moment.

Nothing changed that week.

Some of us made cassette recordings of familiar sounds: the Blue Fountain jukebox, the chimes and clatters of the pinball machines we wasted hours on, even the electronic munching sounds of Pac-Man. We replayed them at his bedside, hoping – praying – that something might call him back.

But nothing changed.

I got the call from Caz, one of his sisters, early on New Year's Day. It was the first day of 1980. Chris had suffered a heart attack in the final hours of 1979. He didn't make it.

After he passed, I left the hotel. The memories were too many, too strong. They used to lift me – make me laugh even when he was far away in Geneva. But now, even the best memories came with an ache. The laughter, once effortless, had a shadow behind it.

The Why

Chris's car collided with a lighting pole outside Blackpool Pleasure Beach. He was heading south, having just dropped the family friend at her hotel, and making his way back to St Annes to join us at the party.

A few hours earlier, the snow had started falling. Not heavy, but steady. Chris wasn't reckless – not when it counted. With a passenger in the car, he'd have been cautious. He would've judged the road, thought it through. If he kept driving, it was because he believed it was safe to do so.

Blackpool Promenade is mostly a straight line – until you reach the Pleasure Beach. There, the road sweeps right and then gently left. It's not a sharp S-bend. It's wide. Easily enough for four lanes of traffic. And it's a 30-miles-an-hour zone.

I went to the crash site. The pole was down, wrapped in police tape. I'd imagined the wreckage being on the opposite side of the road – but it wasn't. That puzzled me.

In the UK, we drive on the left. If you're going straight and lose control in the snow, you'd expect the car to veer left due to the camber of the road surface, not swing across the road to the right and smash into a pole. That kind of movement – almost a 90-degree turn – didn't make sense. Had he swerved to avoid something? Someone?

It happened around 2am on Christmas Day. The lighting pole was still live when his car struck it. Chris's vehicle became part of the electrical circuit. He was unconscious inside, and no one – no paramedic, no firefighter – could touch the car without being electrocuted.

This was the 70s. No mobile phones. Skeleton crews on Christmas Day. It took almost four hours to find someone qualified to shut off the power and get them to the scene.

Four hours.

That's how long Chris lay there, unreachable. Alive, maybe. Alone, definitely.

And yet, when the investigation wrapped, they just...

66

blamed him. No one questioned it. They said it was driver error, and moved on. But it never sat right with me.

The Calypso nightclub was nearby. There would've been a line of taxis on his left. Did one suddenly pull a U-turn in front of him? Did a drunk pedestrian stumble into the road? Something *made* him swerve. I was convinced of that.

Eight years later, on my 29th birthday, I was having drinks with two girls after work in a town you will soon read about. That evening, a touring psychic show was in town. Tickets were sold at the door, and they talked me into going with them.

We sat far from the stage, way up in the circle. The show began with flashing lights and a big round of applause as the medium took to the stage. After his introduction, he paused, looked out at the crowd, and said:

"Andrew? Where are you, Andrew?"

The girls nudged me, laughing. I didn't raise my hand. It's not like I had a name tag. And there were probably a dozen Andrews in the crowd.

Then came the next line:

"It's Christopher! Where are you, Andrew?"

My heart froze.

Christopher. Not Chris. Not the way we said it. We were *Chris and Andy*. But still...

He waited. No one responded.

Finally, he said:

"Andrew, Christopher wants you to know – it was an accident."

I sat still, barely breathing. I hadn't told the girls anything. I hadn't even wanted to be there.

But something in me shifted that night.

For years, I'd carried this weight–the confusion, the guilt, the need for answers. Maybe I'll never know what really happened on that icy road. But maybe that night... maybe that was Chris, giving me a kind of peace.

He's still with me. In old songs, in arcade machine bleeps, in the shared memories which make me laugh and cry at the same time.

Forever in my heart, Chris.

High Flying

Two years into my second architectural practice – you know, the one with the proper salary and the ergonomic chairs which didn't give you sciatica – I did what I always did when life dared to run too smoothly: I panicked at the suspicious lack of catastrophe and promptly quit. No warning. No plan B worth mentioning. I just strutted in, handed in my notice, and declared myself self-employed, radiating the manic confidence of a man who'd had three double espressos and a suspiciously large line of pure hubris for breakfast.

Amazingly – and this is where you might want to sit down – it looked, briefly, like I'd made a genuinely clever move. The two drawing services I'd been secretly moonlighting for squealed with delight when I told them I was flying solo. One even handed me an actual office. With actual walls. It felt terribly grown-up – in the same way handing a toddler a chef's knife feels "grown-up".

Paid per job, the cash poured in like I'd struck oil in my back garden. I was living the dream! Or at least the discount version: no yacht in Monaco, but I was on first-name terms with the bar staff at the fancy pub where the toilets didn't smell like a crime scene.

Sounds sensible, right? To a normal human with an ounce of self-restraint, absolutely. But you know me – self-restraint has never darkened my doorstep.

Have you heard of George Best? (If you haven't, we need to talk.) George was this glorious Irish footballing genius in the sixties and seventies – Manchester United's poster boy before marketing departments knew how to exploit poster boys. Fast, charming, cheekbones sharp enough to dice onions, and a talent so dazzling that defenders wept into their pints long after the final whistle.

And then, dear George did what all geniuses do when showered with cash, fame, and women: he went full Greek tragedy. He made enough money to buy a mid-sized republic before he was old enough to rent a car, so naturally he blew it all faster than it came in – booze, cars, Miss Worlds – until the inevitable tabloid meltdown unfolded in glorious slow motion.

Why mention George Best? Because, my friend, I became the George Best of architectural draughting – except less handsome, with no fan club, and hangovers which could drop a bull elephant.

I knew the cautionary tale. We all did. Did that stop me? Please. If anything, I treated George's downfall as a how-to manual. I went from making a week's wages in an afternoon to racking up three-day hangovers which laughed at paracetamol. Instead of doubling down and building an empire, I took to clubbing on weeknights like I was nineteen and indestructible.

Soon, I was dragging my sorry, pickled carcass out of bed later and later – sometimes my own bed, sometimes the bed of some lovely stranger whose name I forgot before I even found my trousers. Meanwhile, my once-pristine drawing board was gathering more dust than a nun's wine rack.

The drawing services who'd once sung my praises

were now spitting my name like a swear word. Late on jobs, sloppy with plans, still a genius on a good day – but "good days" were rarer than my sober evenings. They eventually did the only sane thing: cut me off.

Overnight, I went from the Next Big Thing to "Who?" in record time.

When I finally reached the humiliating point of not being able to afford a pint – which, in Britain, is the universally recognised sign that you have well and truly cocked up your life – I did the sensible thing. I got another job. Not back at a drawing board, oh no. That would've been logical. Instead, I donned a hi-vis and started grafting in a factory. Because when your professional life implodes, it's tradition to test whether manual labour can crush your soul just that little bit more efficiently.

Did I learn my lesson there? Of course not. I treated punctuality like an optional lifestyle choice, rolling into shifts late or not at all, blaming "alarm clock failure" when in truth it was "too many shots and a questionable kebab at 3 a.m."

Eventually, even the factory bosses tired of my no-shows and polite excuses. So I did what any genius on a death spiral does: found another factory job. If at first you don't succeed, fail in exactly the same way somewhere new – that's the motto, right?

Now, a normal person might see the correlation between drastically reduced income and the need to curb spending. But I, dear reader, have never been normal. The factory pay covered bread and beans but not my champagne tastes – or more accurately, my discount lager tastes at champagne volumes.

I needed a side hustle. Fast. Because if I couldn't feed my bank account, I damn well intended to keep feeding my ego.

A Career Change

My new sideline? Car dealing.

Given my newly catastrophic finances, I started out at what you might charitably call the budget end of the market. The cars I bought were basically one leaky gasket away from the scrap heap, but with some questionable tinkering and a heroic amount of polish, I could just about convince the next unsuspecting soul they'd survive at least as far as the end of the street.

Once I'd flogged a few through the same local paper I'd once delivered (life's poetic symmetry at its finest), I decided to level up. I rented a lock-up – just big enough to squeeze in one car and manoeuvre around it without donating a kidney to a brick wall. It gave me a proper workspace and, more importantly, allowed for a cheeky respray if needed. Spoiler: they all needed it. Thus began my foray into the fine art of automotive deceit.

Around the same time, I moved in with my mate Dave B. We only rented that flat for about eight months, but in that brief, glorious window we transformed it into Party HQ. If the walls could talk, they'd call the police and then join Witness Protection.

It was brilliant. Cheap wine, a revolving door of misfits, and a steady stream of charming young women who – bless them – genuinely seemed to think I was some misunderstood creative genius instead of a hungover ex-draftsman flogging dodgy hatchbacks for beer money.

We lived like playboys – if playboys owned third-hand

Vauxhalls and subsisted on beans on toast. The months blurred together in a haze of booze, bad decisions, and good stories. But in the middle of all that delightful chaos came one moment so startlingly vivid, so weirdly tender, that even my pickled brain couldn't drown it.

One night, halfway through our reign of questionable hedonism, I had the most powerful, freakishly clear dream of my life. And trust me – given my blood-alcohol levels back then, my dreams usually looked like bad CCTV footage with missing frames. But this one cut through the fog like lightning through blackout curtains.

In it, I was standing on the road which runs parallel to my parents' street. I was halfway down, planted squarely on the pavement opposite a family friend's house, feeling weirdly calm and certain something big was about to happen.

Here's where it gets truly odd: from that exact spot, in real life, you physically can't see St Thomas Church. It's hidden behind a barricade of stubborn Victorian terraces – you have to walk two hundred metres south, through the crossroads, then crane your neck to the right at the T-junction before it appears like a postcard.

Yet in my dream, there it was. Towering above everything, the clock face clear as day, like the whole neighbourhood had politely stepped aside for a better view. Not only could I see the church, but right along the side of it – down Clifton Drive with the clarity of an HD drone shot.

Walking towards me was a girl in a pure white wedding dress, practically glowing. She was at least three hundred metres away yet I could see her as clearly as if she were standing right next to me. She held a bouquet at her waist with a grace which made every rom-com heroine look like an amateur. She was gliding towards the church.

Her dress wasn't some princess gown with a mile-long train and six bridesmaids in tow. It was elegant and figure-hugging – silk sash, no frills, classic and impossibly perfect.

Her golden hair brushed her shoulders like sunlight you could touch, topped with a gossamer veil so fine it revealed her features while making her look like she'd stepped out of a Renoir painting.

Her smile was so peaceful, so sure. No nerves, no doubt – just a calm certainty which made my heart clench like an unexpected tax bill. Her eyes – grey with just a hint of blue – locked on mine in a way that told me she knew me completely. Loved me completely. And here's the kicker: I was certain she was coming to the church to marry me.

That was bizarre, because real-life me had always rated marriage somewhere between root canal surgery and a surprise colonoscopy. But there, in that dream? I wanted to marry this woman more than I'd ever wanted anything. I'd have built her a house out of my own liver if she'd asked.

As she drew closer, we locked eyes and moved at exactly the same time – me stepping towards the double church gate, her passing through the little side entrance on Clifton Drive. Our timing was so perfect it felt choreographed by God Himself. And then – just as we were about to meet – the dream slammed shut like a trapdoor.

I woke up bolt upright. The dream didn't drift away like they usually do, turning vague and crumbly. It stayed. Every single detail. Her face. Her smile. Her eyes. The impossible view of the church. It replayed over and over like the world's most beautiful broken record.

I lay there, wide awake, while my brain helpfully looped the whole thing on repeat. Unlike my usual dreams – naked in Tesco, legs made of concrete – this one stuck around like an angelic squatter in my head. It didn't fade. If anything, it burrowed deeper.

Eventually, I emerged from my room looking like a scarecrow who'd lost a bar fight. Dave B, infuriatingly bright-eyed, was already demolishing a bowl of cereal in our so-called lounge-slash-dining room – basically a mismatched furniture graveyard.

He spotted me instantly, eyes narrowing like a bloodhound sniffing out emotional distress. Dave was basically a human lie detector with a minor drinking problem.

"You alright?" he asked, in the tone of a man fully expecting a 'no'.

"Fine," I lied, pouring myself a bowl of suspiciously stale cornflakes – breakfast of champions and failed mechanics alike.

Dave wasn't buying it. He kept watching me like I owed him rent in secrets. After a few minutes of tense spoon-clinking and me dodging questions with the grace of a brick, I cracked.

I told him everything – the street, the impossible church view, the dream bride, the cosmic certainty that I was about to marry a woman I'd never seen in my entire reckless existence.

He listened, face blank, then deadpanned,
"Do it. Find her and marry her. Then the rest of us can have the other women you're neglecting."

Then he cackled at his own joke, slapped me on the back like he'd just cured cancer, and disappeared into his day like nothing had happened.

We never spoke of it again. But I did – in my head. Constantly. For days, the dream looped, her eyes boring into me from some other dimension. It never faded. Even now, if I close my eyes, she's there – a vision so clear it makes me wonder if reality isn't the real dream at all.

At that time, it was a dream which wouldn't go away. Anytime I wanted to recall it, I could, with the same clarity I had when I first dreamt it. But I was going to find out it was part of something which was, and still is, the strangest thing to have ever happened to me. More to come.

Blast From The Past

Eventually, our glorious eight-month lease limped to its inevitable end – vanishing like a tray of Jagerbombs on a Saturday night. We'd done absolutely bugger-all about finding a new place to live. Why plan for the future when you can just wing it and hope for the best? So there I was, back at my parents' house, tail firmly between my legs. Dave, being marginally more organised than a hurricane in a bin yard, landed himself a one-bedroom flat at the eleventh hour. The party was over. Reality was pounding on the door with the enthusiasm of a debt collector and about as much charm.

Selling cars had started as a part-time scheme to scrape together a few extra quid – pocket money to fuel my refined diet of beer and more beer. But after getting heroically fired from the latest production line gig (turns out arriving drunk and occasionally not at all is *deeply unpopular* with management), my side hustle morphed into my main gig. Well – full-time job, part-time commitment. Let's be honest.

Picture my cutting-edge business model, *The Feast or Famine Method of Entrepreneurship.*

I'd pick up some knackered old rust bucket which looked like it had lost a bar fight with a wrecking ball. I'd then spaff my last pennies on paint, parts, filler – maybe even a magic wand. Whatever scraps of cash survived this spree went directly to the pub, where I'd drink myself into a state of blissful denial about my 'career trajectory'. When I inevitably hit rock bottom (again), I'd shuffle back to the lock-up and get cracking.

Most nights I'd be there until dawn, stripping down old motors like I was starring in *Pimp My Ride: Poundland Edition*. Sand, patch, respray – until that sad hunk of metal gleamed like a naked sword. Once it looked halfway respectable – or at least unlikely to give someone tetanus – I'd slap it in the local paper. Boom. Sold. Cash in hand, sometimes within a day. I was annoyingly good at it.

The universe kept tapping me on the shoulder, whispering: *Mate, this is what you're meant to be doing. Lay off the booze. Build an empire.* Did I listen? Of course not. I'm Andy bloody Partington – I treat good advice like I treat early nights: with deep suspicion and outright avoidance.

Maybe it's not that I don't listen. Maybe I just prefer spectacularly terrible life choices.

Anyway – once I had a nice fat wad of cash burning through my jeans like radioactive waste, I'd swagger back to one of the dodgy car showrooms I dealt with. I'd buy another trade-in which looked like it had been used for target practice but which I knew I could drag back from the brink.

Next stop: buy the paint and parts with the glee of a kid in a sweet shop, drag everything back to the lock-up – then promptly lock it up and forget about it. Because, obviously, the pub was calling. Priorities.

This was my cycle: fix car. Advertise it. Sell it. Pocket the cash. Celebrate until broke. Repeat until the liver protests or the bank account begs for mercy. My life:

engine oil and lager, in equal measure.

This carried on with grim predictability until January 1985 – when my world did a backflip so big the Grand Canyon looked like a pothole in comparison. Had you told me a week earlier what was coming, I'd have politely suggested you seek urgent psychiatric help and a nice padded room. Seven days. One monumental twist. My world flipped – and for once, it wasn't because of a dodgy clutch.

It all kicked off a couple of days before a shiny black sports coupe glided onto my sorry excuse for a forecourt. It looked like it had made a wrong turn on the way to a country club. I dealt in rust and regret – this thing was car royalty, polished to within an inch of its life, glinting like a wet seal in a tanning salon. The sun hit its windscreen so hard it nearly blinded me – nature's way of adding a bit of suspense.

The engine cut out. The driver's door swung open like it was headlining at the Palladium. And out stepped...

Damian.

I hadn't clapped eyes on Damian in yonks, but back in the day, we'd muddled through our early twenties side by side. A couple of years ago, he'd pulled off a miraculous career pivot: from full-time benefits claimant and professional layabout to fully-fledged nightclub DJ. Fair play – the lad was genuinely brilliant at it. The sort who could get a roomful of sweaty teenagers waving glow sticks like they were conducting an orchestra for the terminally drunk. Judging by his flashy motor and designer clobber, life had only got shinier since I last heard him bellow "Make some noise!" over a crackly PA. Clearly, he'd avoided the George Best / Andy Partington route of converting sudden wealth into instant bankruptcy.

He parked himself at my table for the classic breakfast of champions – coffee and cigarettes – and treated me to the full saga of his meteoric rise through the sticky-floored world of nightclub entertainment. He did, however, have the nerve to whinge that I hadn't graced his last big gig in Northampton with my glorious presence. As if I'd venture that far from home. My travel itinerary was strictly local: the lock-up, plus every pub and club between St Annes and Blackpool. Basically, a hermit – but with a drinking problem and worse taste in cars.

Then he dropped the bombshell: he'd ditched Northampton for Swansea and was now the resident DJ at *Bonnie Tyler's Nightclub*. Yes, *that* Bonnie Tyler – the gravel-throated queen of "Total Eclipse of the Heart", who could sneeze and hit number one on both sides of the Atlantic back then.

I'll admit it – I was genuinely impressed. The boy had done spectacularly well for himself, and honestly, I was chuffed. I'm not one to begrudge success. I was too busy perfecting my own one-man disaster show to worry about someone else's big break.

Damian carried on moaning about my disappearing act, and fair enough – he had a point. I offered him the world's flimsiest promise: "Yeah, I'll try to swing by sometime," which, translated from Andy-speak, meant "Don't hold your breath, mate." Still, I felt a weird pang of guilt. I never break a promise – and while I technically hadn't made one, it felt suspiciously close.

Truth be told, I didn't even know where Swansea was. Somewhere down south, past the realm of double yellow lines and sensible roundabouts. I knew they had a football team which rebranded from Swansea Town to Swansea City, and apparently they boasted a nightclub owned by a rock goddess. That summed up my Swansea knowledge nicely.

In Trouble Again

The countdown to chaos hadn't started when Damian pulled up in his Batmobile – it kicked off a few days earlier, when I had the distinct pleasure of standing in the dock at our local Law Courts once again. By that point, I was practically a regular act on their grim little stage.

I'd spent so much quality time there that the Usher – the friendly lady who checked in the local riff-raff – greeted me like an old mate.

"Hello, Andy! Back again?" she'd chirp, scanning her clipboard with the dedication of someone who might've made a fine detective in another life.

She didn't even need my surname anymore. Apparently, I was the only Andrew causing enough vehicular chaos to appear in court with alarming frequency.

"Oh, yes – here you are. Court number four today, love," she'd announce, drawing a brisk pencil line through my name as if she were crossing off teabags on a shopping list. Then she'd flash her trademark 'good luck, you idiot' smile and get back to corralling the other local ne'er-do-wells.

Remarkably, she never judged me – that was the job of whichever poor magistrate had drawn the short straw that day.

For the record: I wasn't mugging pensioners or ram-raiding the corner shop. My crimes were purely automotive. If there was a way to break the law with a car, I'd ticked that box: no MOT, no tax, no insurance, no clue. I got pulled over so often the local bobbies probably had my route pinned up on the station wall like a milkman's round.

We were practically on a first-name basis. It was never "Stop! Police!" – more like, "Alright, Andy – what's falling off today?"

They'd circle my car, pretending to look serious while trying not to crack up, then ask,
"Right, Andy. Which bits are we writing up today?"

And off they'd go, smug as you like, scribbling up my ticket while I stood there glowering, quietly seething with that unique rage reserved for repeat offenders of petty motoring crime.

This time, it was speeding: 58 miles per hour in a 30 zone. Not my finest hour – but, to be fair, it could've been a hell of a lot worse.

The two fine upstanding gentlemen who nabbed me for that particular bit of motoring mischief – Martin and Tony – were, by some cosmic fluke, feeling unusually charitable that night. Lucky for me, because I'd just gifted them enough material for an entire season of *Traffic Cops*.

It all began, as these things often did, at a nightclub. When the place finally spat its sweaty, staggering patrons back into the wild, I emerged with a posse of equally wobbly revellers and trudged up the steps to the car park. Parked right at the top – like a spider waiting for flies – was what we affectionately called a Panda car: a bog-standard white Vauxhall Chevette tarted up in police livery, the automotive equivalent of fancy dress.

Inside were Martin and Tony, our local answer to Starsky and Hutch. In a moment of either cocky bravado or total brain fog, I gave them a jaunty wave. They waved back – with all the warmth of undertakers at a funeral.

Parking outside clubs at chucking-out time was standard procedure for the local constabulary. Nothing said "behave yourself" like a Panda car glaring down at you while you tried to remember which shoes were yours.

My own noble steed that evening was a Morris Marina Estate – for anyone not familiar, picture a station wagon clinging desperately to the idea it was worth more than the rust holding it together. It was designed for five people. Making sure we were hidden from sight of the cops, we stuffed in nine. If you're wondering how, the answer is: badly. Elbows, knees, and opinions were everywhere. Personal space was a distant memory – we basically reinvented human Tetris.

Once we'd arranged ourselves into a shape that sort of fit, again I checked for police eyes. From where I was parked, the coast was clear. Off we rattled into the night, the back seat sounding like a rugby scrum trapped in a biscuit tin. Laughter, shrieks, and the occasional creative insult flew around as people's body parts made accidental – or suspiciously deliberate – contact.

Approaching the first passenger drop-off, I clocked a pair of headlights creeping up behind us with that ominous "You're in deep shit" vibe only a copper can emit. It was dark, but every cell in my idiot brain whispered, *Police*.

I barked orders to Jim, the first to be freed from the clown car nightmare. I channelled my inner commando sergeant: "The second I stop, you jump out, leg it inside, and for the love of lager, don't come back out even if the street turns into a war-zone. Got it?"

I hit the brakes. Jim shot out like he'd been fired from a cannon, cleared his garden gate in a single bound, and vanished inside. Door slam. One less human jigsaw piece for me to explain.

Which was handy, because at that exact moment, the mystery headlights rolled to a stop right in front of me. Goodbye dreams of a Hollywood getaway. Hello, Martin and Tony.

Martin unfolded himself from the Chevette and wagged a finger at me – the universal sign for *You absolute muppet, get over here.*

I obeyed. What else was I going to do, floor it with eight people wedged into a car which couldn't outrun a mobility scooter?

He leaned in, deadpan as a tombstone. "How many people are in that car, Andy?"

I gave him my best humanitarian smile rather than a number.

"They're all skint. I couldn't leave them to walk home in this weather, could I?" Because obviously, I was a mobile charitable organisation – Saint Andy's Shuttle Service for the Broke and Drunk.

Martin raised an eyebrow. "Where've you been tonight?"

Well, he'd literally watched me stumble out of Scruples, so a bold-faced lie was off the table. But a bit of creative truth? Always room for that.

"Just popped in for one last pint at Scruples," I said, praying he and Tony had only been parked there for the final few minutes.

Martin almost – *almost* – cracked a smile.

"Funny that. I watched you going into the Queen's Hotel at twenty to ten."

Game over. Slam dunk. Busted so hard my ancestors felt it.

Then came the killer line: "Would you be over the limit if I breathalysed you?"

My entire life flashed before my eyes – mostly a montage of bad decisions set to a soundtrack of beer fizzing and engines dying. But then, by some miracle, Martin's softer side made a surprise cameo.

"I'm booking you for fifty-eight in a thirty. Take that lot home, straight home, and if you get pulled over again tonight – this conversation never happened and you'd better be standing on the steps of the station waiting for me at ten o'clock tomorrow night."

That's when his shift started. He wasn't joking. And I wasn't about to test whether he'd forget.

I took the win. Sure, I got slapped with a £180 fine – not exactly the crown jewels, but enough of a dent considering my next rust-bucket masterpiece wasn't even halfway tarted up yet and my wallet was emptier than a politician's promises. I probably racked up a few demerit points too, but unless they charged interest, I couldn't have cared less.

Pay it on time? Please. I had a rock-solid, six-step strategy for fines:

Step One: Ignore it.

Step Two: Wait to be arrested. They'd usually swing by around 6 a.m. a few weeks later – prime time to catch me at home and mostly conscious.

Step Three: Sit in a cell for a couple of hours, door conveniently open, then enjoy a prison-grade full English which was criminally better than anything I'd ever cooked myself.

Step Four: Be transferred to court at 9:15 a.m. and deliver a heartfelt monologue about my tragic lack of funds. (Pro tip: plead poverty; works like a charm.)

Step Five: Charm the magistrate into a bargain-bin payment plan – a tenner a week if they were feeling generous.

Step Six: Leave court with a grin and enough change left for the pub.

It never failed. Until it did. Because this time, only Step One got a look-in – the rest was steamrolled by what came next.

At that point in my rollercoaster of a life, I technically had a "steady" girlfriend. I say "steady" – but that word was doing the heavy lifting of a medieval siege engine. If you've read this far, you know "commitment" and I weren't exactly on speaking terms.

Her name was Jane – saintly, stunning Jane – who by rights deserved her own chapter in *Hagiography for Modern Saints*. Unlike me, Jane had this quaint notion that truth, fidelity, and paying fines were all, you know... *important*.

To her credit, she didn't glue herself to my hip at the pub. Unfortunately, on the nights she stayed home preserving her sanity, I had a remarkable talent for leaving with an entirely new girl draped over my arm like a living fashion accessory. Don't ask me how – even I couldn't explain that bit of black magic.

Somehow, Jane stuck around. Almost three years, to be precise – which in Andy Partington Relationship Time is basically a life sentence for good behaviour she didn't commit. She was jaw-dropping, the kind of beautiful that made grown men rethink their life choices and fib about everything from age to shoe size just to impress her. Meanwhile, there was me: walking, talking proof that karma sometimes goes on holiday.

Of course, I cheated on her. Of course, I felt terrible about it. And of course, my mates were only too happy to point out what an utter moron I was – they just never mentioned it to Jane, because moral high ground only stretches so far when you fear for your teeth.

Anyway, Jane's big quirk – besides tolerating me – was a flair for catastrophe. She genuinely believed that one day a magistrate would clock my endless encore of unpaid fines, say "Right, enough's enough," and ship me off to an extended stay with Her Majesty's finest. She'd paint these scenes with the drama of a Shakespeare heroine: orange jumpsuit, scary cellmate named Bruiser, my handsome mug gracing the local paper under the words *Serial Idiot Finally Jailed*. I, naturally, found this hilarious.

Still, bless her – she had the patience of a saint and the forgiveness of a golden retriever, provided you didn't push your luck too far. But this particular fine? It drove her up the wall faster than all the others combined. Why? Who knows. Maybe the stars aligned just right for her to lose her last shred of patience.

So, around lunchtime on what should have been a normal weekday, Jane materialised at my lock-up like the ghost of consequences yet to come. This was unusual for two reasons:

1. She couldn't care less about my oil-slick empire, unless her car was on the brink of combustion.

2. Her lunch break was only forty minutes, and she'd just spent half of that getting to me.

To say I was surprised would be like calling the Hindenburg a minor mishap. I half-expected a slap or a break-up speech. Instead, she kissed me – same warmth, zero smile. And Jane's smile was famous: flick it on, and the room went from gloomy pub to Christmas morning. Today? No lights.

She rummaged in her bag like she was defusing a bomb, pulled out a wad of cash hefty enough to make a bookie cry with happiness, and slammed it on my workbench with more drama than an EastEnders finale.

"Go! And pay that f****** fine!"

When Jane used the F-word? You knew you were officially on her last nerve, and things had reached DEFCON 1. This was a woman who said "damn!" When she stubbed her tow and apologised to *furniture* when she bumped into it.

She kissed me again – maybe hoping she wouldn't regret it – then vanished, leaving me alone with my thoughts and a sweaty handful of banknotes.

I counted it like it was the Holy Grail: one hundred and eighty quid, enough to shut up the courts, calm Jane down, and convince my mother I was vaguely responsible. My next move should've been obvious: march to Lytham Courthouse and pay up like a grown adult.

Naturally, my brain said: *Absolutely not.*

See, the breakfasts at St Annes Nick were the stuff of local legend. Greasy, glorious plates of bacon, eggs, sausage, beans, and toast – culinary masterpieces which made you briefly forget you were technically under arrest. Missing out on that? Unthinkable.

So, in what I firmly believed was a moment of genius, I decided to stick to my usual playbook: skip court, wait for the Old Bill to show up at dawn, get chauffeured to the station like a VIP, savour the best breakfast Lancashire Constabulary could buy, and then pay the fine at court with a flourish. Everybody wins.

Feeling smug about my brilliance, I pocketed the cash, skipped Lytham entirely, and headed straight to my parents' place for tea, sympathy, and to kill time until the pub opened.

I'd barely stepped through the living room door before I realised my mother was in a mood so black it could have blocked out the sun. Jane wasn't the only one fresh out of smiles that day.

My mum tracked me from room to room, listing my life's failings with the dedication of an unpaid political opponent. When she got started, she had the tenacity of a bailiff and the stamina of a Tour de France cyclist.

I knew the script by heart:

- *Track One:* "The Drinking!" – a full critique of my beer-based food pyramid.

- *Track Two:* "This House is Not a Hotel!" – a classic, albeit factually inaccurate; hotels leave mints, and my pillow had only ever seen spare change and regrets.

- *Track Three:* "You Were a Fool to Quit Being an Architectural Technician!" – my personal favourite, delivered like a eulogy for wasted potential.

- *Grand Finale:* "Why Jane Puts Up with You, I'll Never Know!" – a question which still baffles scientists and theologians alike.

My parents adored Jane. Worshipped her, really. To them, she was my last, best shot at redemption. In their wildest fantasies, I'd marry her, become a better man overnight, and maybe even hold down a respectable job. Sure. Right after I start bird watching and going to bed at 9 p.m.

I endured Mum's greatest hits for about ten minutes – roughly three Ice Ages in parental argument time – then decided enough was enough. That fine wasn't getting paid today. Five quid of Jane's heroic bailout would never see the inside of a court clerk's till. So, naturally, I did what any rational man would do: I went to the pub.

There, perched at my usual spot, I ordered pint after pint, pondering Mum's speech with all the philosophical depth cheap lager could buy. Somewhere around the sixth or seventh pint, I had an epiphany: maybe she was right. Maybe I *was* a walking calamity. Shocking revelation. Water is wet, the Pope is Catholic, Andy Partington is a mess – news at eleven.

By pint number *lost-count*, I'd hatched my grand plan for a total life reset: But first, I needed a holiday. A proper one. A break from adulting, lectures, and court summonses.

One small hiccup: I was skint. Completely, spectacularly skint.

But wait – not quite! There, tucked safely in my pocket, was £175 of Jane's finest "please-don't-go-to-jail" fund. And guess where that money was about to take me? Spoiler: it wasn't the courthouse.

Croeso I Gymru

The next day found me staring bleary-eyed out the window of a National Express coach, watching the British countryside drift by in that blissful, half-hypnotised, half-hungover state you only achieve when you have no clue how you ended up on a bus to Wales. Yes – Wales. As in, *actual* Wales. This geographical bombshell dropped when we lumbered past a giant brown sign declaring "Welcome to Wales!" in two languages, one of which looked suspiciously like a cat had danced across a typewriter.

Swansea is in Wales? News to me.

The journey was punctuated by pit stops in pint-sized towns which seemed to exist purely so our driver could stretch his legs and remind himself that time, indeed, does pass. People got on, people got off – it was like watching a painfully slow episode of *Coach Swap*. Mercifully, the bus was never full, so I sprawled luxuriously across two seats like I was the Duke of National Express. Best part? I wasn't driving, so there was zero chance of adding another traffic offence to my growing collection. Pure, irresponsible bliss.

As dusk slathered itself across the sky, we rattled into yet another grim bus station which looked like it had been designed by someone who deeply hated buildings, light, and joy. While the driver fiddled with something under the bonnet – or maybe just his patience – I peered through the window at what had to be the world's saddest pub. Lights on, zero customers, atmosphere somewhere between tax audit and dental surgery. The whole street radiated a level of misery which would make a funeral look festive. "Thank Christ this dump isn't Swansea," I muttered, praying to any god who would listen.

A couple more pit stops later – blessedly far from that architectural crime scene – we finally rolled into our final destination. I stumbled off the bus, spine permanently shaped like the coach seat, and barely hit the pavement before Damian appeared out of nowhere and snatched my bag. He looked just as slick as he had back at my lock-up – only now with a slight air of local celebrity. Without wasting time, we made a beeline for The Valbonne complex, his personal DJ kingdom.

The place floored me – like finding a diamond hidden in a skip. Sure, it had that "Hello 1970!" vibe, but it buzzed with genuine magic. Not the plug-in air freshener kind – the electric, people-are-actually-happy kind. Everyone was grinning, laughing, living like they'd just won the Pools. I thought, yeah...I could definitely get used to this.

Downstairs housed the City Tavern (the bar) and the Flambé restaurant (where, presumably, things got flambéed to within an inch of their lives). Upstairs lurked two nightclubs: The Valbonne and Studio 25 – names fancy enough to fool punters into thinking they were classier than the décor suggested.

Damian had the night off because, thanks to ancient dancing laws written by monks or Puritans or whoever hates fun, clubs upstairs couldn't open on Sundays. So instead, we settled into the Tavern for "a few" quiet beers with a crew of locals Damian had already charmed into loyal drinking buddies.

Now, as a seasoned pub dweller, I wasn't exactly new to the art of propping up a bar – but the City Tavern hooked me in ways my beer-befuddled brain couldn't quite grasp. The place was like a warm hug from the universe. The people? Even better.

My first impression of the Welsh? Ridiculously friendly. Warm to the point you half expect them to invite a burglar in for tea before ringing the police. They'll chat with anyone: your gran, your dog, a lamp post if it looks lonely. They've got razor-sharp humour and that accent – dear God, that accent! I could (and still can) listen to Welsh women speak for hours. It's like angels reading bedtime stories – after a glass or two of wine.

For the first few days, while Damian DJ'd his heart out upstairs, I haunted the Tavern and the clubs as the honorary plus-one – golden ticket in hand for free entry and all the cheap lager my liver could tolerate. I was meant to be there for a week, tops. So I resolved to make it legendary. I drank like I was on a mission to dehydrate Wales. I danced like someone with no sense of shame (accurate). I flirted shamelessly – and the best part? None of these lovely Welsh girls had any way to ring up Jane back home.

By the time the week limped towards its hazy conclusion, one thing was clear: Mission absolutely accomplished. And Swansea? It was very quickly stealing my heart.

Should I Stay or Should I Go?

A couple of nights before I was due to leave Swansea and head home, – still pretending this was just a "quick holiday" – I was sinking pints with Gareth, the manager of the whole glorious three-ring circus. Between beers, he asked what my plans were. For reasons even I can't fathom, I said I didn't know. Why I lied is beyond me. I did know: stay a week, stagger back to St Annes, carry on my illustrious career as a part-time car sprucer, full-time bar prop, and occasional visitor to the local magistrate.

Instead, Gareth, in his infinite wisdom (and, let's be honest, mild desperation), said he needed someone to fix a few broken bits around the Valbonne. Apparently, Damian – bless his meddling heart – had told him I was a dab hand with tools and duct tape. So Gareth asked if I fancied earning a few quid. One nod later, I was on the staff. Just like that.

I blitzed every dodgy hinge, squeaky door and drunkenly-kicked-in toilet cubicle within a few days. Job done. Before I knew it, Gareth offered me a bar shift – enough hours for full-time wages and, more importantly, an unlimited supply of free pints. Heaven.

What about St Annes? The lock-up? The half-finished Ford Mustang? The unpaid fine? And, well... Jane? Everything but Jane evaporated quicker than my bar tab on a Friday night.

Jane, saintly and shockingly forgiving, came down for a couple of weekends and even enjoyed herself. Damian – who'd known her back when he still lived up north –

played the gallant host, dragging her on stage so often she practically had a fan club in Swansea by the time she left. I still nipped back home to see her, and we racked up epic phone bills talking nonsense at night, but I couldn't twist her arm to join my Welsh soap opera full-time. Smart girl.

Eventually, I took her to Majorca for ten days as an apology for blowing her fine money on my accidental new life. After that, we split up with minimal fuss. The distance stretched, the calls shrank, and my new flat, in the Uplands area of the city, turned into a revolving door for local lovelies. Even so, Jane stayed the gold standard – gorgeous, sweet, and lightyears too good for me. Was she The One? Close – but not quite. That pint-sized hurricane showed up about a year later, and trust me, she deserves her own scandalous chapter.

Meanwhile, bar life suited me perfectly. The Valbonne was chaos on tap: beer spilled everywhere, floors swimming in lager, tills fit to burst, and tips crammed in my pockets like I was smuggling spare change for Britain. Every shift ended with more cash than sense – plus a healthy stack of phone numbers from girls keen to unravel the mystery of "the cheeky English barman." Spoiler: there was no mystery. Just me, a dodgy accent, and questionable moral fibre.

Then Gareth decided he needed an assistant. Because we drank together and laughed at the same stupid jokes, naturally, he picked me. I wasn't keen. I loved the bar life: hard graft, easy tips, free pints, and daily flirt marathons. Promotion sounded suspiciously like responsibility. But Gareth nagged me sober – a rare feat

– and next thing I knew, I was trading my bow tie for a cheap suit.

In classic Valbonne fashion, Gareth then managed to party himself out of a job. A few after-hours shenanigans caught the wrong eyes upstairs. He was handed his P45 and politely told to jog on. Miraculously, for once, I wasn't involved. I was spending the weekend in the north for my alien siblings wedding. Gold star for Andy!

With Gareth gone, they needed a safe pair of hands. My pair weren't exactly safe, but they were conveniently attached to the only sober bloke in a suit. So in no time at all, I went from clueless handyman to barman to head honcho. Manager, me. And I loved it.

Did Damian have a hand in it? He swore blind he didn't. I remain unconvinced. Either way, we were buzzing. He was the star DJ; I was the boss behind the scenes. Between us, we turned that place into a money-printing fun palace of women, wine, and unrepeatable stories. The St Annes boys were ruling the roost.

Months flew by in a boozy, glittery haze – until HQ decided to clone the magic twenty-five miles away in Bridgend. Same owners, same Bonnie Tyler rubber stamp, and one upgrade: Damian was now on the board. Our rock 'n' roll empire was expanding.

Trouble was, Valbonne Bridgend was doomed before they even hung the sign. It opened Thursday, Friday, and Saturday nights, but punters preferred closer clubs in the town centre which didn't require oxygen tanks to scale a giant hill. Back in its glory days, the building – then called Drones – was the only show in town. Now it was just inconvenient cardio with a disco ball.

Three months in, the poor sod they'd hired to run it was canned. The directors wanted a saviour. Translation: they wanted *me*.

I loved Swansea. My team worked their arses off and I adored every one of them – from glass collectors to bar staff to doormen, we were a family of reprobates who got the job done. For the first time ever, I felt like I *belonged*. So when the summons came to "pop upstairs for a quick chat," I did the sensible thing: I bolted.

That didn't work. Their offices were just two floors above mine. They gave up waiting, marched down to my office, barricaded the door with a director, and boxed me in like a suspect on *Crime Watch*.

Keith, the senior director, opened with a grin wide enough to power Swansea, which I made disappear faster than Lord Lucan.

"Andy, you're the new manager of Valbonne Bridgend."

My reply was both elegant and professional: "Like *fuck* I am."

Cue ninety minutes of bribery and flattery. Every ten minutes, they upped the offer: more cash, perks, the moon on a stick. What they didn't grasp was that I wasn't angling for a raise. I just really didn't want to abandon my Swansea madhouse. Honestly, I'd have paid for my own beer if that is what it took to let me stay.

But, as always, good sense lost out to relentless pressure. After ties were loosened, the last round of bribes hit the table, and my will to argue dissolved. I caved.

On February 28th, 1986 – after a rowdy, teary send-off which still gives half my old staff a misty look after a few pints – I fired up my wheezing car, merged onto the M4, and pointed myself east.

Bridgend was calling. A failing club. A steep hill. And a fresh mess with my name on it.

Valbonne, Bridgend

On my first night at Valbonne Bridgend, I didn't know a soul – not even the staff I was supposed to be managing. I stood in the foyer trying to look authoritative while flanked by my two doormen, who regarded me with the warm trust one usually reserves for dodgy insurance salesmen.

One of them was a towering six-foot-six slab of muscle named "Tiny," obviously named by someone with a sense of humour and a death wish. The other was barely taller than the doorknob and answered to "Little Peter," which, to be fair, fit him down to the shoelaces.

I didn't hang around for polite introductions. Tiny attempted to chat, but he had a stutter so ferocious that by the time he'd wrestled the first syllable into submission, my mind had already wandered off to more pressing matters – like, *Why the hell did I say yes to this place?* For all I know, Tiny might still have been trying to finish his sentence when I sloped off to meet the rest of my new crew.

At least Damian had agreed to come down and apply his DeeJaying skills every Saturday night for my first three months – a lifeline for a venue on life support. But that first Thursday? Seven customers. Seven! I had more staff on shift than punters on the dance floor.

Friday night crawled up to a glorious ninety. Saturday limped to a whole one hundred and twenty. I could've made more money selling warm cans of lager door-to-door in a retirement village. The grim reality hit me like a hangover: I'd traded a goldmine in Swansea for a ghost ship on a hill. Brilliant move, Andy. Truly inspired.

Still, despair and I had an understanding: I'd let it knock, but I rarely invited it in. So Monday morning, I rolled up my sleeves, squared my shoulders, and declared war on empty dance floors. I threw everything I knew into promoting the place. I headed into town and charmed local businesses and hospital staff by day, doling out stacks of free entry tickets like some budget Willy Wonka – except instead of chocolate, the golden ticket was a guaranteed hangover.

Whenever I handed tickets to the pretty ones, I sweetened the deal: *"Find me when you get in – first drink's on me."* Cheap? Maybe. Effective? Absolutely.

Meanwhile, on Saturdays, Damian had a system: he'd kick off the night by blasting a cassette tape through the PA, then vanish into town to tour the pubs, handing out more free tickets and hyping the place up like a carnival barker on bonus commission. Free entry was no bother – the real money was in the rivers of vodka and pints once we got them inside.

Four weeks later, the Marie Celeste had become a floating riot. More than twelve hundred bodies squeezed through the doors on Fridays, with Saturdays matching them pint for pint. Even Thursdays were bouncing. Technically, the fire code said the place could hold four hundred and fifty people. We may have slightly... exceeded that. If the Chief Fire Officer had swung by, he'd have needed a paramedic and a stiff drink. Oops.

Bridgend's Valbonne was roaring – and, mostly, it was

down to me. The directors were convinced I was the second coming, a manager with a Midas touch and no regard for occupancy limits. I even printed myself a tongue-in-cheek pass that read: *Andy Partington: Allowed To Do Whatever The Hell He Likes.*

One Friday night, in the middle of the chaos I'd created, I was pushing my way from the lower bar to the upper bar – no easy feat when the entire population of Bridgend seemed to be grinding against each other under your roof.

Halfway through the sweaty crowd, I stumbled on something odd: a clear patch of floor, a neat little no-man's-land about three or four square metres wide. In a club so packed people were practically dancing on the ceiling, an empty spot was more suspicious than a priest at a poker game.

I glanced at the carpet. No puke. No broken glass. No sign of a fight or a forgotten handbag. Just empty floor, ringed by baffled gyrators.

Then, like Moses parting the Red Sea, the revellers opposite shuffled aside, and through the gap stepped a young blonde with that dangerous glint only Welsh girls seem to perfect. She planted herself squarely in the clearing, gave me a look which could melt steel, and asked, in that sing-song accent I'd come to love:

"Are you the manager, then?"

God help me – I had a feeling my night was about to get very interesting indeed.

Dream Dream Dream

I genuinely don't know how long I stood there like a broken coat rack. From the outside I must have looked like a bloke who had simply forgotten how to function.

She was... devastating. Eyes the colour of storm clouds threatening to ruin your BBQ – mostly grey, but with a sly flicker of blue. And that half-smile she gave me? Nations have fallen for less. There she was – flesh and blood – the actual girl who'd been renting space in my subconscious for FOUR BLOODY YEARS give or take. In my dream, she'd been wearing a wedding dress. In reality? She didn't need a veil – she was dressed to kill, and my heart was the first casualty.

So there I am, drooling, brain whirring like a dial-up modem from the 90s. She goes, *"Are you the manager?"*

I panicked. "YES!" I barked. Probably loud enough to startle the next county.

Then she hits me with: "Got any bar jobs going?"

Did I? Not unless I fired some of the staff and replaced them with houseplants. We were fully staffed – standing room only behind the bar.

But my mouth had other plans: *"YES!"* I croaked, like a man rediscovering the joy of lying on the spot.

The conversation was short but we agreed she'd start the very next night. She sashayed off, probably telling her mates she'd just scored a job from some moron in shiny shoes. And me? I just stood there, blinking at the mass of bodies she'd disappeared into, asking myself if

I'd just hallucinated the last five minutes.

Normally, after closing, I'd buy my staff a pint, do a bit of gossip, maybe a cheeky singalong if the mood took us. That night? Forget it. They could drink my share. I parked myself at the far end of the bar, pint in hand, rewinding that dream in my head like it was my favourite soap.

Was I losing the plot? Had I deepfaked my own dream girl into existence? Was this the same girl? And if so – HOW? Truth, I didn't care. She was real. She was drop-dead gorgeous. And tomorrow night, she was going to be mine. Well... behind the bar, at least. Let's not get carried away.

The next day dragged. I did the usual nonsense: cellar checks, beer lines, cash floats, all the mundane stuff which comes with running a nightclub. But my mind wasn't in it. It was spinning, locked on NJP – which is what I'll call her here, because real names get messy in court.

How was it even possible to dream about a girl you'd never met – and then meet her years later and recognise her instantly? I'd watched that dream more times than I'd watched *Only Fools and Horses*. I was constantly checking my watch. I was starting to think the evening would never arrive. Time actually slowed down – I swear it.

But eventually, 8.30 p.m. rolled around – and there she was. Punctual. Immaculate. A walking distraction in a white blouse, tight black trousers and a smile which should've come with a health warning. I threw her on the busiest bar in the club – sink or swim, sweetheart. Sink or swim. I told myself, *"No favouritism, Andy. Be professional."* Then I immediately begged every god I could think of to please, please let her swim like an Olympic dolphin.

I watched her the way David Attenborough watches a rare snow leopard: silent, hidden in the shadows, completely entranced. She was glorious. She poured pints, mixed spirits, handled cash like she'd invented the concept – all while throwing that smile at punters so dazzling they forgot they had wives at home.

I was so deep in my lovestruck stalker routine that I didn't even notice one of my regulars sidling up next to me. He clocked my gaze straight away – fair play, it wasn't subtle. He told me he knew her – then he casually detonated my entire night:

"You do know she's sixteen, right?"

Sixteen! Six-bloody-teen! My stomach hit the floor so fast it left skid marks.

Silence.

So not only was she behind my bar illegally – I was basically running a child-labour speakeasy. Was I a responsible adult who immediately fired her on the spot? Absolutely not.

Anyone else? I'd have chucked them out the fire exit mid-pour. But her? No way. She could've told me she was twelve and I'd have rung a lawyer for loopholes. (Okay, not twelve. I'm creepy, not criminal.)

I let her finish the shift – sue me. I needed to think – which, trust me, was a radical new concept for me.

I knew I had to take her off the bar. She was underage, I already had staff on coat check – and keeping her on risked a knock on the door from the licensing cops, and given the existing arrest warrant floating around from St Annes for "failure to pay fines", I wasn't exactly keen on more quality time in a courtroom.

How do you sack the girl of your dreams *without* losing her forever? Invite her out for a quiet drink to explain? Oh sure – twenty-seven-year-old boss invites sixteen-year-old girl for a secret pint. That's not weird at all. Even I knew that was a one-way ticket to a tabloid headline.

So I did what I had to do. When the lights came on, the drunks were being slung out, and the bar smelled like stale lager and broken dreams, I called her up to the office.

She didn't lie. Not for a second. Just stood there – big eyes, innocent face – and owned it. Sixteen, knew the law, sorry boss. I gave her my best fake grown-up lecture about fines and prison (which was hilarious given my own record) then said exactly what my heart was screaming:

"You're bloody brilliant at this. The second you turn eighteen, I want you back behind one of my bars."

Then I watched her cute backside disappear through my office door – and I swear I aged about ten years in that moment.

DIY and NJP - The Sequel

Over the next few months, my life turned into the plot of a very low-budget sitcom. By day, I was supposed to be a nightclub manager. By night... also a nightclub manager. But in between? Full-time handyman, part-time electrician, occasional plumber, and unofficial marriage counsellor to a set of toilets which refused to stay unblocked for more than twelve hours.

The Valbonne, Bridgend – my pride and recurring ulcer – had been refitted in record time and for princely sum of what seemed to be the price of a pint and a bag of crisps. Everything looked shiny enough on opening night, but within a week it was basically held together with duct tape, crossed fingers, and my increasingly colourful vocabulary.

So when the owners of a brand new mega-venue – 'Aston's' – popped up and offered me the chance to run it, I didn't exactly ask for a written contract and three rounds of interviews. It took me approximately two seconds to blurt, **"Yes, please dear god get me out of here."**

Of course, there was a catch. There's *always* a catch. Aston's existed solely on fancy planning drawings and the fever dreams of its investors. It wouldn't be ready to open for at least a year. But no problem – I'd just keep babysitting The Valbonne until Aston's was built, then waltz across town in a blaze of glory like the Pied Piper with my current customers in tow. Easy.

Except... not.

Barely had I rehearsed my triumphant exit when word came down that The Valbonne's lease (along with me) had been flogged off to a national nightclub chain. They were planning yet another refit (good luck with that) and to do it properly this time, they were shutting the place for months.

And me? Well, the plan was to pack me off to run *another* one of their clubs somewhere else in England. Which sounds fine – except I was really starting to like Bridgend. I'd found my groove, made actual friends, and – most importantly – I was completely, hopelessly, absurdly obsessed with the idea of bumping into NJP again.

I mean, come on – how many people can say they've literally met the girl of their dreams? She'd been haunting my subconscious for years before waltzing into my bar like she owned the joint. And then, poof! Vanished with nothing but her name and the memory of her smile, which I replayed nightly like an old VHS tape.

No address. No number. She was underage, so it's not like I could just find her propping up the next bar along (legally, anyway). And let's be honest – after hiring and firing her in the same night, I was the last bloke she'd be dropping a CV off with.

So, faced with the prospect of being shipped off to the arse-end of nowhere by my new corporate overlords, I did what Andy Partington does best: I quit. I stuck around Bridgend, picking up part-time bar shifts and lurking in every local pub like a romantic stalker with an overtime addiction. If NJP was out there, I was going to find her. Or drink myself into believing I had.

A year later – after enough planning meetings, builder bust-ups, and budget crises to age me a decade – we opened the doors of the pub and nightclub in a frenzy of bright lights and publicity. The venue was an instant success. So much so, the club upstairs opened at 9 p.m. but the queue was forming by 8:30 – snaking around the block like people queuing for free gold.

I'd never seen anything like it. I'd also never worked so hard. In the weeks before launch, I'd been on a one-man reconnaissance mission disguised as a boozy pub crawl. The goal wasn't to get wrecked – although I heroically failed at that part spectacularly – but to scout the best bar staff in town and poach them for my dream team.

And poach I did. If you could pour a pint without crying, you were hired. If you could smile and multitask, I begged you to join. By opening night, I had a crack squad behind my bars.

All except the one I really wanted.

NJP.

In twelve months of combing every watering hole in Bridgend, I never saw so much as her shadow. Nobody I asked knew her. There was no Facebook, no Instagram – just me and my stubborn faith that she'd appear again, like a glitch in the Matrix.

Then, on a Friday night ten days after opening, it happened.

I had closed the pub down at 11 p.m. clearing out all the customers who had just parted with their hard-earned with the help of my team of doormen. Upstairs was bouncing and before I headed up there to mingle, meet and greet, I decided I would have a moments peace and a cigarette.

I cracked open the side door of the pub again, just enough for a lungful of icy Welsh air. The bass pounded through the floor above me – *Thud! Thud! Thud!* The DJ was doing what DJs of that time did best - bang out enough volume to try and blow the PA system off the wall. But somewhere over the top of the auditory mayhem, I heard stilettos clacking on concrete.

Curious, I poked my head out of the door. Two young women in short skirts were strutting up the opposite pavement like they owned it.

And then my heart did something truly stupid. It stuttered, stammered, and tried to crawl out through my throat.

The one on the right was NJP.

She was right there – hair bouncing, eyes everywhere *but* me, pretending she hadn't clocked the idiot gawping at her from a doorway. I watched and waited for the right moment.

When they drew level, I couldn't help myself. I called out.

"Oy!" Simple but effective.

"Hey, Andy! Didn't see you there!" she lied. Of course she had seen me, but I'm guessing she still thought I was pissed off at her for the Valbonne incident. She would have had no idea how pissed off I was, but not at her, at the law which kept her from me.

She crossed the road like she hadn't spent a year living rent-free in my head. She was more stunning than ever, all dressed up for a night on the town – not a hint of bar uniform in sight.

She had remembered my name. My heart did a backflip.

I didn't even glance at her friend (rude, I know – sorry, love). All I cared about was NJP, standing there under a streetlight, looking like a wish someone had whispered straight into the universe's ear.

I cleared my throat, channelled my inner responsible adult (which didn't take long, because he barely exists) and asked:

"You eighteen yet?"

She smirked. "Nearly."

"How nearly?"

She cocked her head. "A few weeks."

I shook my head dramatically.

"You are eighteen. You had your birthday two months ago. Congratulations. You're rostered on tomorrow night. Eight o'clock sharp."

For a split second, I braced myself for a rejection. She could have laughed. Told me to shove it. Walked away forever.

But instead – she smiled. The same smile which had launched a thousand daydreams and exactly one illegal hiring incident.

She didn't have to say yes. Her grin told me

everything.

I flicked my cigarette, strutted back inside, and punched the air like a twelve-year-old whose crush had just agreed to hold hands at the disco.

Sure, she was still underage but not by much – minor detail. If the licensing cops found out, I'd have some explaining to do. But in that moment, with the music blasting and the dance floor heaving, I didn't care. She was worth doing prison time for.

Paul's Casino

The following day, while I pretended to manage a pub and nightclub, my mind was about as present as a ghost on annual leave. It looped one word: NJP.

I'd barely glimpsed her on nights out – apart from that unforgettable evening she strolled in and turned my heart and my employment policies upside down. So I didn't know: was she the kind of girl who got so hammered she'd wake up convinced she'd hallucinated me? What if she'd forgotten she'd agreed to come back and work for me?

I paced, fussed over stock levels, and checked the tills five times. Then, at 7:45 p.m. on the dot, she walked in. Ready for work. Same dazzling smile. Same effect on my vital organs.

Her first night at Aston's was déjà vu: she poured drinks faster than physics allows, weaponised that smile on every punter in reach, and made me look like a competent manager. What more could I want? (Don't answer that.)

One perk of running a pub and nightclub: you're a kid in a sweet shop which never closes. I lived with my head doorman, Paul – a walking brick wall with fists like dinner plates and a matching attitude. Like me, he was single and tragically weak for pretty faces and bad ideas.

Between us, we drafted an unofficial house policy: *No one goes home alone if there's an alternative.* Every weekend, a fresh parade of party girls tagged along after closing time, eager to keep the night alive – in every sense. There were occasional repeat visitors, but mostly it was a revolving door of *'good fun, nice to meet you, let's never discuss this in daylight.'*

Routine was simple: Paul's crew cleared the dance floor, I cashed up, and by the time the last drunk was taxi-bound and the bar staff clocked out, our guests of honour lurked in the shadows, waiting for an after-party which made the tabloids look tame. To our knowledge, only my assistant manager knew the full extent – and he was on a strict need-to-know diet.

We thought we were discreet geniuses. Spoiler: we weren't.

You're probably wondering: How does a guy juggle all that bed-hopping and claim to adore NJP like some tragic poet? Excellent question. Here's the truth: I was a fucking idiot.

In my deluded head, the wedding scene from my recurring dream meant she and I were inevitable. But until I figured out how to get her alone – not as a barmaid, but as a date – I clung to my adolescent playboy fantasy. After all, nobody really knew, right?

Whenever NJP was on shift, I transformed from Playboy Andy to Pathetic Puppy Andy. I'd leave my office under the noble pretence of *checking in with staff* – mostly just to stand too close to NJP and talk nonsense about ice buckets and till shortages. Embarrassing. I was embarrassing.

Once the music swallowed my excuses, I switched back to Mr Charisma: leaning on the bar, chatting up customers, and deploying lines something like – "Hi, I near as damn it own this place, want to see my sofa?" Miraculously, it worked.

If I found a willing candidate, I'd discreetly signal Paul, who handled the exit strategy like a bouncer-cum-escort service. We thought we were pulling off Mission Impossible every night. In reality, the only girl who lived rent-free in my daylight thoughts was NJP – but I had no clue how to upgrade awkward stock talk to an actual date like a functioning adult.

The last real relationship I'd had longer than six hours was with Jane – and I couldn't remember how I'd managed that. I'm fairly sure, relationships in the past just happened to me: no plan, no depth, just vibes. With NJP, I wanted more. Much more. But short of tattooing *Please love me properly* on my forehead, I was out of ideas.

So, naturally, being Andy Partington, I made it worse. I complicated everything by occasionally sleeping with a couple of the barmaids – purely one-night stand material, of course. My assistant, James B, ran interference. He wasn't the world's greatest club manager, but he was brilliant at mopping up my mess before it exploded.

Ask James B his job title and he'd smirk:

"I follow Andy around cleaning up his carnage."

He wasn't wrong.

Since my barmaids and NJP got on well, poor James basically lived on high alert for the next nuclear love triangle. Somehow, he kept the powder keg from going off – but only just.

On Sunday, by law, the pub shut at 10:30 p.m., the club stayed dark, and if Paul and I didn't hit an all-night Little Chef for a late night breakfast, we usually made it home by midnight – sometimes alone, more often not.

One Sunday, though, I skipped the chaos and promised myself honest sleep. I was knackered and needed it. Paul had set up a poker game in the 'Casino' – his converted garage turned adult playground: pool table, darts, bar stocked like Aston's. It was legendary among our crew: Paul's Casino, where fortunes vanished before daylight thanks to dodgy shuffling and too much booze.

A few doormen and local taxi drivers grabbed seats at the table. Me? Not a chance – my poker face leaked like a sieve, and my wallet had suffered enough. As the guests began to arrive, I cracked a beer for politeness, wished them luck, then, as the deck was being shuffled, I retreated into the house for what I thought would be a quiet night.

And then the universe, forever amused by my plans, did something totally unexpected...

Heaven or Hell

I'd just flopped into bed, on the brink of switching off my bedside lamp, when my door begun to creak open.

At first, I figured it was one of the poker maniacs stumbling around hunting for the bathroom. I was mentally preparing to grunt directions when the door swung wide – and my entire nervous system threw in the towel.

Time froze. My heart might have stopped altogether, though not for long enough, clearly, because it immediately slammed back into overdrive. For a second, I wondered if I'd dozed off mid-reach for the lamp and drifted into a dream. But no – whatever this was, it wasn't a dream. Trust me, I'd become an accidental expert at telling dreams from reality.

Reality, however, was struggling to explain this one. Maybe I'd just died and an angel had arrived to collect my battered soul – destination to be determined later, based on available vacancies in Heaven or Hell. Odd thing was, this angel looked suspiciously like NJP. Exactly like NJP, in fact.

The door stood wide open and there she was, standing in my doorway, beaming like I'd personally invented the sunrise just for her. My brain short-circuited. She hadn't been anywhere near the house when I escaped the chaos downstairs. If she had been, believe me, I wouldn't have come up to bed alone like some monk on a detox retreat. I'd have been glued to her side, inventing urgent bar stock emergencies to justify breathing the same air.

From what I've pieced together – and trust me, piecing this together is like solving a murder with more than half the clues missing – she might have turned up with Paul's new girlfriend, Anna. Paul had bolted from the pub earlier, in a mad rush to get everything 'perfect' to impress his poker guests, leaving Anna to find her own way back to the house. NJP must have tagged along for moral support, wandered into the poker room, clocked the high stakes and testosterone stench, and decided she was better off out of it.

Why she didn't just leave altogether, I'll never know. But instead, she stepped inside my room, quietly closed the door behind her, and sat herself down on my bed like it was the most natural thing in the world.

My heart was pounding so hard it probably left bruises on the inside of my ribcage. And then I did what any idiot in my position would do: I pulled back the covers and invited her in. Anyone else, I'd have done it with cocky confidence, figuring the worst they'd do was giggle and leave. But with her – oh, no. This was everything. For a second, as she hesitated, I thought I'd just detonated my one chance with her forever.

She sat there, staring at me. An eternity stretched out – though in real time, it was maybe two seconds. Then she spoke: no sex tonight. Just sleep. Did I care? Absolutely not. Having her that close was better than anything my usual antics ever delivered. She might not have been an angel sent to ferry my soul skyward – but that night, I was definitely in Heaven.

There are moments in life you recognise instantly as turning points: telling Batman "we're done here"; walking into the City Tavern for the first time; hiring NJP in the first place. Her getting into my bed was another of those seismic shifts. Everything was about to change – and for once, I was fairly sure how it would unfold.

I was a nightclub manager living in a beautiful house (technically Paul's, but details). I got paid decent money to drink, smoke, and misbehave with women who, in hindsight, deserved better. By day, I pretended to run a business; by night, I partied like I'd invented 'rock and roll'. To any single guys watching, Andy Partington had it all.

But right then – with NJP pressed against me, her warmth seeping into my bones, her soft Welsh lilt wrapping itself around my heartbeat – *this* was having it all. Everything I'd ever secretly wanted since the moment she'd stepped in front of me in The Valbonne, demanding to know if I was the manager, was lying right there in my arms.

Her breath fluttered against my chest, her blonde hair brushed my cheek, and her right hand rested over my heart, fingers rising and falling like she was playing a lullaby on my ribs. I was cocooned in a happiness so pure I almost didn't recognise it: undiluted, terrifying, perfect.

We didn't move. We barely slept. We just talked – a conversation I'd waited for so long I sometimes doubted it would ever happen. She admitted she'd always had a thing for me, but there were two giant, mother-shaped and Andy-shaped reasons she'd kept her distance.

121

First: her mother's iron grip on her romantic choices.

I'd met NJP's mum when she organised a *Tarzanagram* for her daughter's eighteenth birthday at the club. As you can imagine, watching a semi-naked man in a loincloth swing into the pub area and announce, *"Eighteen today!"* was only slightly less mortifying for me than for NJP. The staff pretended they hadn't just learned our angelic barmaid was actually still a baby in club years. NJP, however, was humiliated. Apparently, she'd once confessed her crush on me to her mother, who responded by verbally obliterating her: no way was her daughter going near that older man.

She'd listened. Of course she had. Meanwhile, I'd been too busy playing nightclub Casanova to notice she'd been right there, crushing quietly behind the bar.

Second: the parade of women I left the club with every weekend.

To this day, I have no idea how she knew about every one of them. Paul and I thought we were stealth ninjas. Turns out we were about as discreet as a conga line. She even knew their *names* – which is more than I did. Mid-conversation, she'd mention *"So what about Zoe then?"* and I'd have to stall: *"Er... which one was Zoe again?"* It was humiliating but I deserved it.

As the sun threatened to rise, she admitted the real kicker: she'd come to the house that night because she knew I was alone. How did she know that? God knows. Probably the same telepathic network she used to catalogue all my other dalliances.

In my head, that admission was it: we were about to

be official. The moment she crawled under those covers, I saw my new life flicker into life: First thing in the morning I would go to the club and hand in my resignation with immediate effect. I wanted marriage, kids, a mortgage, Sunday morning lawn mowing, a sensible estate car, an utterly boring nine-to-five so I could spend my evenings and weekends with her. I was ready. I wanted it all more than I had ever wanted anything in my entire life.

And then, like the romantic genius I was, I said the quiet part out loud: something about us being a proper couple.

Instant. Cosmic. Error.

I watched the beautiful, Technicolor dream in my head drain to black and white in seconds. NJP gently, firmly told me it was never going to happen.

Excuse me, what? Hadn't she just crept into my bed? Told me she'd fancied me? Crossed town in the middle of the night to lie here, wrapped around me like a cat claiming its favourite warm spot? My brain spun in circles.

She explained: she liked me – *liked me! liked me!* But she wasn't going to waste her sanity wondering every night if I was out bedding half of South Wales the minute she turned her back. And fair enough, I suppose – my track record didn't exactly scream "trustworthy future husband." But the tragic twist was: with her, I knew I would have been different. I would never have cheated on her if we had lived to be a million years old.

As she laid it all out, my panic bubbled up. Had I

misread this whole night? This whole night which I considered to be the best night of my entire existence. Was this some sort of payback for being a walking disaster? Did the two barmaids I'd treated like disposable party favours team up with NJP to expose me? Was this her plan – get me to spill my lovestruck guts, then torch what little respect I still had among the staff by telling all and sundry what I had told her?

My paranoid minuscule brain kicked into gear. If she was going to blow up my world, maybe I needed to strike first. Protect the scraps of dignity I had left. If I was going down, I was taking every angel down with me.

Betrayal

The following morning, I did something wildly out of character: I turned up at the club *early*.

On Mondays, my assistant always clocked in before me to tackle the grim realities of cellar work – swapping empty barrels for full ones, sorting the graveyard of empty bottles for the brewery's recycling run, and restocking the bars to fuel the next wave of chaos.

Normally, I'd breeze in halfway through, pretend to care about stock rotation, then vanish to drink tea whilst spinning excuses about 'managerial paperwork.' But that morning, I grabbed a barrel and actually helped. Why? So I could keep an eye on him *and* steer the gossip before it blew up in my face.

It was rare for me to confess anything about my extracurricular activities – discretion being the only thin veil covering my disastrous reputation – but I told him I'd spent the night with NJP. I even told him we didn't have sex. If we had I would have not been in the cellar, I would have been in the office with the directors handing in my resignation.

To throw him off any possible scent of scandal, I sprinkled in a few tasteless jokes at her expense – painting it like a regrettable blip I'd never repeat. Brutal, yes, but necessary, or so I thought. Should any whispers circulate – and trust me, whispers always circulated – he'd have a version ready to muddy the waters. Mission accomplished, I left him rattling barrels and returned to my office to bask in the shame of my own betrayal.

Sitting alone, I replayed what I'd done. Christ, did I really think NJP would run to the bar staff and announce we'd snuggled all night, and I had confessed my undying love for her, like a teenage rom-com? The paranoia which had driven me to poison her reputation – and mine – was pathetic. By midday, I'd accepted what my heart had been screaming since dawn: NJP wasn't a gossip, wasn't a manipulator, wasn't a revenge plot in stilettos. She was the one person who had never given me a reason to doubt her. And I'd repaid that by pre-emptively throwing her under the bus to protect a reputation which wasn't even worth saving.

The morning after our night together, she'd slipped away in a taxi. And deep down – somewhere under the bravado and self-pity – I knew she'd never come back. Not to me, anyway.

By the afternoon, I'd cycled through shame, regret, and a few fantastically doomed daydreams in which I apologised so eloquently that she'd sweep back into my arms forever. Spoiler: she didn't.

Only hours before, I'd been wrapped around the most beautiful woman I'd ever known – not just in my bed but in my future, in my daydreams of kids and mortgages and dull Sunday chores. That single night remains the best night of my life. And yes: I didn't get the girl, but I got perfect recall. Even now, I can close my eyes and feel her breath on my chest, her fingers tapping that quiet piano rhythm on my ribs, her hair brushing my jaw.

What terrifies me most – far more than any health scare – is that one day I might forget the tiny details: the way her voice softened in the dark, the warmth which

126

made the rest of my life feel colder by comparison. I'd trade half my memories to keep those few hours vivid.

Love you, NJP. Always. xx

And so, life bumbled on – minus the after-hours harem.

I quit the post-closing pick-up routine cold turkey. Within days, Paul and Anna were convinced I'd caught some unspeakable venereal plague. Paul cornered me in the lounge at home, demanding to know *which* STD I'd contracted and whether he needed to quarantine the bathroom.

After I convinced him I was disease-free, I confessed the real reason: NJP. I admitted everything – how I felt about her, what had happened, how I'd spectacularly cocked it all up. To his credit, Paul didn't laugh, didn't judge, didn't even try to sell tickets to the drama. He promised he'd take my secret to the grave. And, bless him, he did. RIP, Smudge – the only bouncer who could break a nose and keep a confidence in the same night.

Secretly, I hoped NJP would somehow notice I wasn't leaving the club arm-in-arm with some giggling stranger anymore. Maybe she'd see it as a sign I'd changed. Maybe she'd forgive me. Maybe she'd give me another chance.

She didn't. And not long after, she found someone else. A bloke I knew and liked, too – which somehow made it worse. I was gutted, but what could I do? Chase after her screaming *"Pick me, I'm reformed!"*? I had to take the loss like a grown man – or at least pretend to.

A couple of months later, I left the club altogether. One of the regulars offered me a sales job and, honestly, I needed a change of scenery. Seeing NJP with her new guy felt like slowly peeling a plaster off a wound which never healed. Plus, one of the directors had started poking his nose into the day-to-day running of my kingdom, acting like he'd invented nightclub management – despite never having run so much as a lemonade stand.

I wasn't in a good place. Murdering him seemed increasingly reasonable. For his health and my criminal record, I decided to bow out gracefully instead of throwing him off the roof balcony.

Years rolled by. I heard NJP had married, had a couple of kids, did everything I once imagined doing with her. And yes – it still stings. Sometimes, late at night, I catch myself fantasising: I hear a knock, open the door, and there she is, ready to run away with me at last. It's pathetic, romantic, tragic – all of it. It's never happened. And even though sometimes I still run the fantasy, I doubt it ever will.

After her, I changed – mostly. I stopped the conveyor belt of one-night stands. Another friend, Nikki T, who is partially responsible for this book, once summed it up best: no woman worth her salt could ever trust the old Andy Partington to be faithful. She was right. NJP knew that too – and she made her decision accordingly.

From that time on, I swore I'd only sleep with women I was in an actual relationship with. And for the most part, I kept my word. (Disclaimer: I'm not a saint – there were a few slips between relationships. Old habits die harder than my pride.) But in the main, I tried to become a better man. For her. Even if she never saw it.

I didn't get the ending I wanted. But I got the night I needed. And if that's all I ever get from NJP – it's enough.

Back In The Car Trade

Going back to a nine-to-five after the madness of nightclub life was like stepping out of a hurricane into a tepid puddle. Suddenly, I had evenings free – which sounds wholesome until you remember I'm me. I could have taken up crochet, or adult education, or yoga. Naturally, I opted for the only logical thing: I went to the pub.

My new boss – or should I say ringleader – was John, a gloriously unhinged Irishman who owned the car yard I'd somehow found myself flogging used motors in. He was as unpredictable as a cat on cocaine, which made him equal parts hilarious and infuriating. Like me, John didn't just "enjoy" a beer – we both regarded it as a food group. Conveniently, we lived near each other in Bridgend, so we often stumbled home together to the symphony of his wife's disapproval.

It turned out I was still good at selling cars and I regularly had John's rivals sniffing around, trying to poach me like I was some sort of prized truffle pig. John and I argued constantly – the kind of rows where the windows rattled – but ten minutes later, we'd be back at the bar, pint in hand, as if nothing had happened. Work stayed at work; the pub was sacred ground.

After a couple of years, I caved to one of the offers which seemed to be coming my way almost constantly and jumped ship for another sales yard. Over the next eight years, I bounced around four different places – new cars, old cars, lease deals, you name it. I was selling dreams on four wheels with a smile and zero shame.

Then the universe fancied upping the drama in my life and reintroduced me to Ellen. I'd hired her when I was running the Valbonne in Swansea. She'd come up to Bridgend for wild nights out and somehow, and I genuinely can't pinpoint when, she simply... didn't leave. One weekend visit morphed into her moving in. One day, she was my guest; the next, she was arguing with me about the bathroom lightbulb.

"Turbulent" is the polite word for what we were. We argued about everything and nothing, usually after enough vodka to embalm a horse. She'd scream, I'd shout, she'd slam the door and hop the train back to Swansea, vowing never to see me again. Give it a week, one drunken phone call later, and we'd be back at it – the row, the train ride, the explosive make-up sex – rinse and repeat like a tragic soap opera no one asked for.

One Friday in August '95, we did what we did best: got obliterated. I woke up the next morning with the sun scorching my retinas, the curtains wide open, and Ellen beside me – so I knew at least we hadn't had a row bad enough for a midnight flounce.

And out of my vodka-fried brain popped this gem:

"What are you doing three weeks from today?"

"Dunno. Why?" she mumbled.

"Fancy getting married?"

Honestly, I've never seen someone evacuate a bed faster without a fire alarm. She shot out the door so quick she left her clothes in an unapologetic heap on the floor,

131

probably terrifying the neighbours as she bolted down the street half-naked, leaving me blinking at the ceiling, wondering if I'd just imagined the whole thing.

Moments later, though, I realised she hadn't left the house. I heard her chattering at warp speed on the phone to her mum. Turns out the answer was yes. So, we did it. Got hitched. And true to my hopeless romantic core, I half-hoped NJP – the woman I really loved – would burst in during the "speak now or forever hold your peace" bit, declare undying love, and rescue me from my own idiocy. She didn't. So instead, we got merrily drunk at the reception, as tradition demanded.

Life bobbed along nicely for a bit. We bought a cottage in a postcard-perfect village on the edge of Bridgend – which looked quaint until the walls practically fell off. The surveyor clearly had cataracts. Long story short: we had to bulldoze and rebuild the entire thing. But convinced Cefn Cribwr was where our happily-ever-after would happen, we rolled up our sleeves and got it done.

Around that time, I landed a sweet gig in car leasing. As an extra carrot, they gave Ellen a company BMW even though she didn't work for them – she loved rocking up to her mates' houses pretending she was Lady Muck.

Then came 1999, when, for reasons lost to the mists of drunken pub chat, I decided to see a medium called Zena. Just for a laugh.

On the day of my reading, Ellen "called in sick" at her own place of employment and tagged along to my workplace instead – the first time she'd ever done that. In hindsight: suspicious.

Zena didn't mess about. For a whole hour, she gave me a blow-by-blow of my future. At the time, I thought half of it was mystical waffle, but over the next twenty years, every word unfolded exactly as she'd said – right down to the cancer she cryptically hinted at.

Early on she kept repeating, "Look after your wife." I thought, Great, she's got the flu or something. Nope. Turns out Ellen was having a grand old affair with "Smiler", one of her Swansea buddies. Zena had obviously seen it swirling in her crystal ball and given me the only clue she could without handing me divorce papers on the spot.

Once the dots joined up, I was more bemused than enraged. Ellen had always been my plan B, if I'm honest. If life had been fair, NJP would have been Mrs. Andy Partington. So, when Ellen finally picked Smiler over me in February 2000, I put on my best wounded-hero act – just in case she fancied crawling back – but truth be told, I didn't want her to. She deserved her happy ending.

Time To Go Home

In the strange limbo between my ill-fated chat with Zena, the psychic, and Ellen pulling her Houdini act with Smiler, I did what any self-respecting man would do to keep his sanity: I threw myself back into the twilight world of nightclubs and pubs.

Back managing a club and pub open until the early hours when, in reality, I preferred a quiet pint and a kebab by eleven.

I had agreed to help out a friend who was having a few problems with staff so he got me to go in and root out the problems.

Working late nights made it easier for Ellen to hop in her car and slip down the M4 to Swansea for a bit of illicit romance with Mr. Smiles-A-Lot. She'd always tell me she'd had a quiet night in, watching some soap or other, but the car's mileage never lied.

It wasn't even detective work on my part – just a half-hearted glance at the odometer whenever she tossed me the keys. She never twigged. To this day, she's blissfully convinced she outfoxed me. According to her, I think she left for her soulmate in one clean break and I never suspected a thing. Well, surprise darling – if by some cosmic joke you're reading this now: yes, I knew. But no, I didn't care enough to confront you. I was too busy serving pints to drunks, and dreaming about a woman I actually loved.

The club I was running at the time Ellen packed up her toothbrush and affection was called Monroes –

named, of course, after Marilyn, who, much like me, had an unfortunate taste in lovers. The company who owned it also ran Jaggers (Mick, not knives), Taylors (Elizabeth, not shoes), and a few other celebrity-inspired watering holes scattered around Bridgend. We were the Poundland version of Hollywood nightlife, but the punters didn't mind.

Monroes was like Astons in its heyday: local pub on the ground floor, chaotic club upstairs where every bad decision made perfect sense under strobe lights and a sticky ceiling. Fridays and Saturdays, the place throbbed with sweat, hormones, and the smell of spilled cider. There were so many bodies crammed in that I could barely keep track of the staff, never mind the punters.

Years later, I discovered that NJP – yes, her again – used to come to Monroes while I was running the joint. The love of my life, dancing ten feet away, pint in hand, while I sat in the office daydreaming about her like an idiot. She never once told a bouncer or barmaid, "Hey, tell him I'm here." Not once. And finding this out twenty years later still stings more than I care to admit.

But why would she? She probably never knew what she meant to me. How could she? I didn't have the guts to say it the one night we were alone. I planned to. God knows I planned to. But I let my own tangled mind convince me I wasn't good enough. And so she danced in my club, unseen, and walked away every time.

Funny side note – remember back in '85, when my hungover soul rode that National Express to Swansea, stopping in a grim little town I moaned about for a whole paragraph? I peered out into the night and spotted a sad old boozer called The York Tavern, looking like it had given up on life. Well, slap on a bit of paint, add a neon sign, and voila: The York Tavern became Monroes. Back then, I'd never have guessed I'd one day run the place under a new name.

Bridgend transformed from a dump on a detour to the place I called home. How could it be anything else? It was the scene of my greatest memory – even if the girl I should have been with never knew.

Fast forward to April 2000. Ellen was gone. Smiler had his prize. The cottage was emptier, the dog bowls were still full, and my pride was somewhere under the sofa. So, in an uncharacteristic moment of clarity (or maybe insanity), I decided it was time move on.

I grabbed my two dogs, a battered suitcase, and a few belongings I thought I couldn't live without – mostly a half-dead plant, my favourite mug, and some old photos I probably should have burned. I loaded up the car and pointed it north. Back up the same roads I'd come down fifteen years earlier, only older now, and maybe – just maybe – a little wiser.

As I wound through the Wye Valley's green dreamscape, sunlight flickering through the trees like some film director's final flourish, memory after memory flicked through my mind like an old slide projector: the nights in Astons, the chaos of Monroes, the fights with John the Mad Irishman, the laughter, the benders which turned into confessions, the mornings I wished I hadn't survived – and always, like a stubborn heartbeat in the back of my skull, NJP.

I thought about how the Welsh – these loud, kind, stubborn, fiercely loyal people – had taken in an Englishman with more baggage than sense. They gave me laughter, drink, friendship, and fights worth having. They let me belong, even though I was a stranger. Wales is, was, and always will be God's Country in my eyes – no cathedral ever made me feel as blessed as the sticky floors of a packed pub in Bridgend or Swansea on a Friday night.

But for all that warmth, for all the gifts Wales gave me, it also gave me a ghost I still carried. NJP – the dream I conjured into reality for one perfect night, the one who never knew, the one I'd have torn down the stars for if she'd only asked.

So there I was, driving away with my dogs snoring on the back seat, waving a silent thank you to the hills and valleys which had forgiven so much of my madness – and wondering, with a sad smile and a heart still stupid enough to hope.

Why did life give me the one thing I wanted most, only to snatch her away before I even said the words?

The Prodigal Son Returns

I was still on the fence about how I felt returning to St Annes after fifteen years of pretending it no longer existed. My family still lived there, as did a good handful of old friends, though most of them now had mortgages, toddlers, and back problems, so the chances of finding them out on the piss were slim to none. Aside from blood relatives and half-forgotten mates, I couldn't tell you what else had changed in town – I hadn't paid much attention the first time around.

But here I was, back again. And I knew one thing for certain: staying in at night was never going to be an option. So the mission was simple – choose a new local. Or rather, revisit an old one and hope it hadn't turned to shit in my absence.

My first notion was to head back to "The Vic" as it was known locally.

The Victoria Hotel, designed by John Dent Harker, was built in 1897 and opened for business in 1898 in honour of Queen Victoria's Diamond Jubilee. It was an outstanding piece of architecture. Years before, when I stood out the front, I could imagine that back in its heyday, it oozed luxury. There was space forward of the front door where the horse-drawn carriages would have pulled up and guests would have alighted, able to take in the opulence of the new majestic building before them. In my imagination I could see them ascending the entrance steps as the carriage slipped away to the left before turning towards the stables at the rear of the building.

By the time I became a regular in 1976, the hotel's Downton Abbeyness had faded into its dotage. Inside, the once lush carpet had been replaced with budget oil-based linoleum, which bore the holes of much passing trade. A darling trip hazard if ever there was one, though not a health and safety issue back in the day. Not everyone was trying to sue the arse off everyone else so health and safety hardly existed. Should you have tripped as you strayed into the vicinity of curled-up floor covering and spilt the entire contents of your pint glass, or broke your leg, it was your fault for being careless! Go back to the bar and buy another one, or go up to the hospital and get fixed. DO NOT go back to the bar and gripe about it! Simpler rules for simpler times.

The wallpaper which had survived the passage of time, although discoloured and water stained, peeled and hung away from lime-plaster walls which also bore the holes of negligence and decay. What once appeared to be inches thick varnish had long since been rubbed away from the elegant, mahogany doors and staircases.

All in all, apart from the immaculately kept snooker table in the games room, the whole place was in serious need of a tad more than some gentle, tender, loving care. But as regulars, we didn't give a monkeys chuff about all that. Why? Because the beer was outstanding. Boddington's Bitter at its finest and *nobody* did it better.

It wasn't just beer back then. It was a religion. Pulled by hand from the freezing cellar by a local barmaid whose right bicep could crack walnuts. The swoosh of it flowing into a glass – oh, I can still hear that heavenly hiss, even now. A pint cost next to nothing, so you could spill half of it and nobody cared. Wipe your chin, buy another, get back to the gossip.

Deliveries were an art form. Enormous oak barrels, each the size of a baby elephant, eased off the drayman's wagon with all the care of a heart surgeon. Then came the delicate ritual of rolling it down rails into the cellar, cradling it for two days so the beer could calm its nerves before being unleashed on the public.

Norman – 'Bleedin' Norman' to his fans – ran the place like a monastery. He wouldn't tap a barrel before its time, even if every punter in town was baying for blood. Quality over profit, always.

And what a taste! Before preservatives and corporate mergers ruined everything, Boddington's was nectar – a pint so smooth it made lesser beers taste like dishwater. Over time the oak barrels gave way to shiny aluminium kegs and chemical stabilisers, the soul was siphoned out along with the sediment.

Back in the day, beer in oak casks only had a travelling limit of around 50 miles, but by the early 2000s, you could fly a pint halfway round the globe – I proved it by ordering one in Australia – but the taste had about as much character as an airport lager. Progress, apparently.

So, there I was, meandering through the streets of my old stomping ground, looking forward to enjoying a few pints in the dilapidated, yet quaintly reminiscent of a bygone-era, pub.

I strolled through Beauclerk Gardens, a small area of lawns with a central shelter pointlessly sheltering nothing but pigeons. The gardens were the immediate neighbour of The Vic. Once across the manicured grass, the hotel was front and centre in my view. I crossed the forecourt filled with excitement assessing the facade of what felt like an old friend.

The red Accrington brickwork, associated with many of the hotels, schools and train stations built in the same era, still wore its grime like a private investigators Macintosh. The Tudor beams and plaster were still waiting expectantly for another coat of paint which should have been delivered more than one hundred years before. It was just how I left it.

My pace quickened. My hand eagerly pulling at the old entrance doors which, as I remembered, required an extra amount of effort to combat the self-closer attached to the top. I stepped inside. My eyes adjusted. My heart cracked.

What the F###?????

The outside may not have altered during the last century, but the interior had been butchered beyond all comprehension.

The small snug little rooms with sporadic wonky chairs and tables? Gone! The exquisitely detailed mahogany staircase which had once elevated guests to their rooms? Gone! The torn and lifting linoleum? Gone! The bar across which I had conducted thousands of pounds worth of money for beer trades? Gone! And some clown had painted just about every wall green. And I don't mean that pastel shade of green which scientists have deemed the most calming and relaxing colour in the history of the universe. No! I mean green as in potting shed green. The same green used to camouflage a Sherman tank in a swamp!

The new bar was brightly lit and the staff poncing around behind it were clad in striped uniforms which made it look more like Nando's than a pub of historic importance! This would never do!

With the wind taken viciously out of my sails, I stepped back across the threshold, released the door handle, and let the over-enthusiastic door closer smash the door back to its resting position. The door and its closer were the only things which hadn't changed, though neither had been spared by the idiot painter.

I retraced my steps back across the forecourt with a lot less vigour than I had when I approached. What was I supposed to do? Accept it, re-enter, and try not to think of yesteryear?

No! With my sensibilities irked, I quickly concluded a visit to the Queensway would be in order. Or perhaps that too had been subjected to modern designer destruction also. Did it now resemble a MacDonalds or maybe a seven-eleven. There was only one way to find out.

The Queensway

During the awkward interim between my sudden departure and equally sudden reappearance in St Annes, my parents had done something which felt borderline betrayal: they'd downsized. Gone was the roomy house just off the town centre where I'd scuffed every skirting board and hidden contraband under the floorboards. Now they inhabited a neat little two-bedroom bungalow so far towards the outskirts I half-expected to see cows grazing the front lawn.

It wasn't all bad though. The Queensway Pub and Restaurant lay conveniently around the corner from the new parental nest – a practical detail which might yet make this homecoming tolerable. Assuming, of course, that the passing years had either fogged memories or removed them altogether. If so, I could nurse a few pints in peace until the ritual cry of "Last orders at the bar, please!" forced me to wobble home like a respectable grown-up.

Mind you, this optimistic plan depended entirely on a favourable resolution to the dilemma I'd been mulling over during the brisk fifteen-minute stroll from The Vic. The last time I'd graced The Queensway with my presence – which back then fancied itself the poshest watering hole in town – I'd been not-so-gently *invited* never to return.

Well, I say *invited*. The reality was a stream of expletives so rich it would've made a sailor blush, delivered at such volume and velocity that spittle rained into   the air like confetti at a wedding I hadn't RSVP'd to.

In fairness, the Landlord's creative tirade wasn't reserved solely for my benefit. I'd been accompanied by Bernie – my co-conspirator, partner-in-pints, and fellow "public menace." Apparently, we both qualified for permanent blacklisting.

And so, as I trudged towards my possible doom, I did the maths. Over two decades had dribbled away since that memorable brawl. My hair style had changed dramatically i.e. less of it, my middle had advanced i.e. more of it, and even my mother claimed she barely recognised me these days. Would the staff or regulars spot the miscreant beneath the middle-aged façade? Would the same landlord still rule the roost with the same frothy vengeance? Or had time carried him off to some celestial beer garden?

I crossed the car park, boots crunching on loose gravel, and allowed myself a fleeting nostalgia trip to *that* night – the night my reputation and several tables met untimely ends.

It began innocently enough: two blokes on motorcycles, leathers squeaking, helmets under arms, dreams of a quiet pint or two after a spirited ride. No one told us that our mere presence would provoke a certain breed of regular – the type who believed any man in leather must be an unwashed reprobate, just a gear-shift away from tearing up the car park.

First round: uneventful. We drank. We chatted about nothing. Life was good.

Second round: attempted, but thwarted by a well-aimed shoulder barge courtesy of a local hero.

One push led to another, which led to fists, which led to someone discovering that a motorcycle helmet could be weaponised with startling efficiency. There was a lot of punching, more than a fair share of broken glass, and at least two tables which learned the hard way they weren't built to withstand sudden disassembly.

And yet – and this is the hill I'll die on – *we didn't start it*. We just finished it. Hands down. Or, more accurately, fists up.

After we'd made our point and made some enemies, we left before anyone had time to call the local constabulary. Or so we hoped. The landlord, red-faced and vibrating with rage, planted himself in the doorway to issue a parting promise: if we ever set foot in his establishment again, he'd personally beat us senseless. Odd how he hadn't joined the melee himself if he was so confident in his pugilistic prowess.

Anyway, here I was, twenty years and a receding hairline later, about to test whether grudges truly mellow with age. I caught myself wondering about Bernie – my co-brawler. Where had life thrown him? Had he settled down? Grown respectable? Or met the inevitable fate of too many road warriors – a wreath on a roadside and a half-remembered name?

These were thoughts for later. For now, I reached the Queensway's door and, like a teenager about to sneak into a nightclub with a fake ID, I peered through the restaurant window first. It still looked up-market, all polished brass and tasteful fairy lights – fancy enough that spilling your pint would feel like a mortal sin.

I wrapped my fingers around the door handle and ran through possible scenarios like a cautious gambler weighing lousy odds:

Worst case: The same landlord, same spittle trajectory, same shouty exit – but with a side order of ageing bruisers seeking revenge in the car park.

Slightly less worst case: He's not there, but his faithful regulars are – and still itching to finish what we started.

Best case: Nobody recognises me. I sip a pint, enjoy my nostalgia, and walk home under the stars, dignity intact.

My personal code dictated that if it came to a fight, I'd get stuck in early and give it my best shot. If defeat loomed, I'd sprint like a champion athlete carrying a bag of stolen gold. Age has taught me a few things, after all.

Taking a steadying breath which didn't feel nearly steady enough, I pulled open the door. I hadn't taken two steps inside when the universe decided to reveal its cards.

"F###### hell! Andy Partington! As I live and breathe!"

The voice boomed out like a cannon in a cathedral. I froze mid-step, part terror, part surprise – and then I saw him: Bernie. Older, softer around the waist, but unmistakably Bernie, grinning from behind the polished bar like a king surveying his loyal realm.

In that moment, two questions answered themselves:

1. I would not be leaving in a flurry of fists and insults.

2. Bernie, my brother in pub-based crime, was very much alive – and now, miraculously, the landlord of the very pub we'd once nearly dismantled.

I'd bet my last pint that our little incident hadn't come up during his job interview. And as he waved me over with the same mischievous glint in his eye he'd had all those years ago, I knew two things for certain:

I was about to enjoy the most satisfying pint in twenty years. And I'd better pace myself – I had a feeling the night might turn into a very, very long story indeed.

An English Country Garden

Bernie landing the landlord gig at The Queensway was an unexpected jackpot for yours truly. Within days, I'd been absorbed into his merry band of regulars – a far less judgy crowd than the frosty brigade I'd previously encountered in that same establishment. The beauty of regulars is they're, well, *regular*. And as a man who considered pub-hopping a noble hobby, Bernie's crew guaranteed me conversation, laughter, and more excuses to nurse a pint or five every evening.

It didn't take long before I forged some solid, beer-bonded friendships – chief among them was Kerry H, who, whether she likes it or not, must shoulder some blame for this very book you're holding. Kerry didn't actually live nearby, but her mum and her sister Hayley did. Hayley worked behind the bar at the 'Q', pouring pints and tolerating drunks with saintly patience. Whenever Kerry came up to visit family, she'd pop down to the pub and park herself on *our* side of the bar with me and another new reprobate in my life – Stevie G.

Relax, Liverpool fans. No, *not* that Stevie G. I hadn't suddenly stumbled into the company of football royalty – our Stevie G was a year my senior, had been a fixture of St Annes since birth, and somehow we'd managed never to cross paths. We never worked out how that was possible, but once we did meet, we wasted no time making up for lost years. Firm friends instantly – bonded by beer, bad jokes, and a shared knack for doing sod all on a Sunday.

A couple of weeks into my triumphant return to St Annes, I found myself on a gloriously warm Sunday evening strolling over to the Q with the Old Dear and the Old Man in tow. The sun was shining, the birds were chirping, and the beer garden beckoned. We parked ourselves at a picnic bench, and I barely got my first mouthful of lager down my gullet before my mother launched into her favourite hobby – *interrogating her only son about his life choices*.

Yes, there'd been a faint whisper about me maybe running a pub down in Neath, just outside Swansea, but that plan had collapsed faster than my last relationship. Undeterred, Mum pressed on with her third degree – oblivious to the fact our glasses were screaming for refills. So, off I trotted to the bar to preserve the family peace.

I returned like some mythical hero – two fresh pints and an orange juice balanced expertly in my hands. I plonked them down and, feeling brave, asked Mum what she was quizzing me about before I'd legged it inside. She picked up right where she left off.

"Oh that," I said, in my best casual tone. "I've got a job. Start tomorrow."

If you've never seen your parents struck mute, I highly recommend it. They stared at me like I'd sprouted antlers. Five minutes prior, I'd been a feckless, unemployed layabout. One quick dash to the bar later, I was still a layabout – but now a *working* one. Magic.

The real magic trick? How I'd blagged it in the time it took to pour a couple of pints.

Turns out, as I sidled up to the bar for the refill mission, I bumped into Martin – another new face from Bernie's circle. Following pub etiquette, I greeted him with the obligatory, "Alright, mate? How's things?" – expecting the usual polite lie in return.

If Martin was ever going to lie, it wasn't going to be on that day.

"Pissed off, if you must know!" he barked, loud enough to silence the fruit machine.

Before I could back away, Martin unloaded a rant at machine-gun speed. He ran a gardening business and employed a couple of local scallywags who'd just texted to say they couldn't be arsed coming to work on Monday morning. He needed someone reliable (tick), someone who could drive (tick), and someone who'd show up on time (tick – as long as I didn't sleep through my alarm). I admitted I knew bugger all about gardening but swore blind I'd learn fast. He shook my hand. Boom – gainful employment, courtesy of a beer run.

And so, I spent that glorious English summer wielding a mower. When the weather played nice, it was the best job in the world: mowing lawns, chatting nonsense, leaving neat gardens and happy punters behind. And the pay? Just enough to keep me in Bernie's good books – and his till ringing every night.

When the skies inevitably turned traitorous, Stevie G roped me into his side hustle: a bit of carpet fitting, and a whole lot of handyman work for locals who paid cash – which, by some mysterious force of nature, always found its way back over Bernie's bar.

Then, as 2002 dawned with all the promise of a fresh start, Ellen – my soon-to-be-ex – popped up wanting to make it official. No point in dragging it out, I thought. I suggested she toddle off to Swansea courts, grab the forms, fill them in, and post them my way. I'd scribble my name and ship them back. No lawyers, no drama, no point scoring. She probably wanted to marry Smiler anyway – the same Smiler she'd been doing star jumps with behind my back for years.

By April, a solemn brown envelope told me I was legally single again. No fanfare, no sad violin. Just me, a steady supply of beer money, and a giant question mark: *What the hell am I going to do with the rest of my life?*

Perth, WA - Part 1

Over the previous year – mostly between the ungodly hours of midnight and dawn, after stumbling home from the pub far too cheerful to sleep – I'd struck up an online friendship with a girl called Rebecca. She lived in Australia, of all places, and turned out to be dangerously easy to talk to, especially when I was propped up in bed with a can of Stella and an existential crisis. She shared my daft sense of humour and tolerated my tipsy ramblings, which, in my book, made her practically a saint.

So, when I broke the news about my shiny new status as a free man – the ink barely dry on my divorce papers – she asked the question everyone else had asked too: *What next?*

Well, in the eighteen blurry months leading up to my unexpected return to bachelorhood, Stevie G and I had been living like part time smugglers – weekdays at The Q, weekends on the Costa Brava. A local guy we both knew owned an apartment out there and, being the generous soul he was, happily funded our EasyJet tickets. The only catch? We had to smuggle, sorry, *carry,* five thousand cheap Spanish cigarettes back home on each trip. The Spanish sun, cold San Miguel, and a cheeky tax-free profit – what could possibly go wrong?

Everything, when your glamorous Mediterranean escape turns into a glorified cigarette mule service. Eventually, it started to feel less like a weekend away and more like unpaid work for the mafia. So, when Rebecca asked where I planned to run off to next, I decided I'd have a proper break – somewhere far from Spain, far from nicotine, and preferably full of sunshine and laughter.

She didn't just suggest Perth, Western Australia – she actually invited me to stay with her. It probably took me about thirty seconds to weigh up the pros and cons (Sun? Tick. Warm welcome? Tick. Possible romance? Tick, tick, tick) and another five seconds to type, "Put the kettle on, I'm coming."

Flash forward a few weeks and I was on a 747 lifting off from Manchester Ringway Airport, clutching a miniature Shiraz and a smug grin. Somewhere over Germany, I remembered Zena's prophecy. She'd told me, three years prior, "I see you heading off to Australia... or even further!" At the time, I'd laughed her off – back then I was flogging cars for a living, not exactly raking in Air-miles. But there I was, 38,000 feet up, Singapore Airlines feeding me wine and movies, and suddenly her words felt less like psychic nonsense and more like a prophecy coming true.

I thought back to a few more of her cryptic messages. *Who's the girl with all the hair?* she'd once asked, as if I kept a secret harem of shampoo models. My mind had jumped straight to Dawn F from Bridgend. Dawn was gorgeous and I had spent a good part of 1990 with her. If you remember the Cher music video from "Turn Back Time", filmed on an American warship, you will remember the amount of hair Cher had at that time. Dawn's was not dissimilar. But striding through Perth Airport arrivals, sweaty and jet-lagged, I clocked Rebecca

153

standing there – and dear God, her hair made Dawn look bald.

After more than a year of digital banter, there she was: in the flesh, beaming, and with more curls than a shampoo ad. We hugged like old friends – or maybe like two people slightly terrified they'd catfished each other – and within an hour, she'd spirited me away to Scarborough Beach.

By sundown we were ensconced in the Stamford Arms, clutching pints of Boddingtons, laughing at absolutely nothing, and ignoring the world until the bouncer reminded us the pub was closing and we needed to leave before we fused to our chairs.

The next month? Bliss. Rebecca would vanish most mornings to play responsible adult at the hotel where she worked as a Duty Manager, and I'd wander the local coffee shops nursing a mild hangover and pretending to read a guidebook. When her shift ended, she'd rescue me and off we'd go – beaches, parks, hidden gems I'd never found online because my travel research consisted mostly of searching "best pubs near me."

Rebecca took my half-baked tourist list, laughed at half of it, then replaced it with places she *knew* I'd actually enjoy – and she was always right. Somehow, despite never having breathed the same air until then, she understood me better than people who'd known me for decades.

The days were bright, the beer was cold, and I don't think I stopped laughing once. My phone's camera roll filled up with selfies of sunburn, sandy feet, and

Rebecca's unstoppable mane of hair blowing in the breeze.

But here's the thing about perfect months – they fly by at breakneck speed. One moment I was landing in Perth, grinning like an idiot; the next I was back at the airport, hugging Rebecca goodbye and trying not to look like a complete sap.

Standing in that departure lounge was the single worst moment of the whole adventure. Not the twenty-hour flight back, not the impending British drizzle, but *that* goodbye. My face ached from smiling for a month straight, and I'd have given anything to rewind it all and do it again, day by sunny day.

As the Boeing 767 banked over the Western Australian coast, I watched Perth shrink away beneath me – blue ocean, tiny roads, endless bushland. Would I see her again? Had she enjoyed it all as much as I had?

Her email landed a few days later: yes, she'd laughed just as hard. Yes, she'd cried as she watched my plane vanish into the blue. And yes, finally – blessedly – she could get a decent night's sleep now that my midnight chattering had flown halfway back across the planet.

Perth, WA - Part 2

Stevie G met me as I passed through the arrivals lounge at Manchester Airport. I hadn't expected him to be there, we hadn't made any arrangements for my return. I didn't want him to be put out if I did what I did when I turned up in Swansea. Went for a break and stayed for fifteen years. He rocked up out of kindness "just in case".

That same evening, as if I'd never left, we were perched on our familiar stools at The Queensway, each with a pint in hand, soaking up the comfort of routine. But the bar felt darker somehow – not because Bernie had forgotten to pay the electricity bill, but because my eyes had been spoilt rotten by a month of blinding Australian sunshine, blue skies, and technicolour everything. Now, I was back to northern England's ambient gloom and suffering from the emotional free-fall which physics warns us about: what goes up must come down, usually with a thud and a hangover.

For the next couple of years, I busied myself with renovation jobs – the odd leaky ceiling here, a bathroom renovation there – until a bigger adventure came knocking. Our Kid had mates in the South of France who owned a sprawling house they'd ambitiously decided to "do up" but couldn't find anyone who wouldn't scarper halfway through the wallpapering. Through Our Kid's backroom diplomacy, I landed the gig. So I stuffed most of my tools into my battered car, pointed it south for Dover, and bounced over the Channel on the ferry, ready to dazzle the French with my distinctly British building site swearing.

My new digs were the actual house I was renovating – a rambling old pile in Tournefeuille (try saying that after three pints), the second largest suburb of Toulouse. Living on-site had its perks: no commute, free bed, and daily practice of my *ahem* schoolboy French.

Back at King Teds, I'd scraped through French O-level with just enough vocab to ask for a postage stamp and a train ticket – handy for a GCSE exam, but about as much use on a work site as a waterproof towel. What I needed were the French words for "drywall", "screwdriver", and "where's your nearest B&Q?". Oh, and cigarettes, obviously.

At the time, France had strict rules: cigarettes were only sold in state-run "Bureaux de Tabac". Every few days I'd shuffle into the one nearest the house and attempt to mime "Benson and Hedges Silver" while butchering their beloved language. The poor woman behind the counter – an uncanny doppelgänger of my terrifying primary school headmistress – endured my garbled attempts with saintly patience and possibly an internal laugh track.

To her credit, over time she started throwing simple questions my way, probably to stop me just grunting and pointing. As a result, my sentences grew from tragic to passable. My "umms" got shorter. Some days, if I managed a full sentence without turning red I'd walk out feeling like Gérard Depardieu.

On my last day, I popped in to say goodbye – in my best French, of course. She smiled, wished me *au revoir*, and then, in the crispest Queen's English you've ever heard, said,

"Your French has come on a treat during your time here."

Touché, Madame. Touché.

When I was in the town centre and wasn't charming French tobacconists, I was gawping at local estate agents' windows, mentally redecorating other people's houses. Property seemed dirt cheap compared to back home. I even found a run-down twelve-bedroomed chateau with fourteen acres of land for half a million Euros. Half a million! In the UK, that might have got you a semi next to a chip shop. I seriously wondered: should I buy it and spend the next decade transforming it into a boutique hotel?

But every time I pictured that château, Rebecca popped back into my head. Even after my holiday, we'd stayed close. At first, we stuck to Messenger, then graduated to long phone calls – well, *she* did the calling, because Telstra made it dirt cheap for Aussies, while BT would have billed me like I was phoning the moon.

Over all those calls, it turned out we both suspected this thing wasn't just mates bantering across hemispheres. We wanted more time, real time, without a looming return ticket. At first, we hatched a plan for Rebecca to come to the UK – she could swing a year-long work visa thanks to her ancestry. But somewhere in the paperwork shuffle, that plan did a U-turn. It was decided: I'd head back to Perth.

During that glorious first month together, we'd been

almost inseparable – beach walks, aimless drives, hours sprawled on towels swapping stories and sand. Not once did we lapse into awkward silence; if anything, we probably gave the seagulls tinnitus with our constant chatter. So we figured: what's a better test of compatibility than living together in the blistering Aussie heat with no easy escape route?

I applied for a Fiancé Visa. The rules were clear: I could live and work in Australia, but within nine months, I'd better either marry her or scarper back to Blighty – or risk being frog-marched to the airport by Immigration with a polite "Cheerio, Mate!"

So, on New Year's Eve 2004, I landed back in Perth on a one-way ticket, full of optimism, romance – and big plans to party with the Aussies and toast in 2005 in true local style.

To ensure I didn't disgrace myself by falling asleep mid-celebration, I thought I'd have a quick power nap before we headed out.

I woke up in 2005.

Wedded Bliss

The wedding wasn't happening until July, so naturally we took our sweet time planning it. We agreed on a small, tasteful affair – no ice sculptures, no doves released at the vows, just a handful of witnesses and enough wine to keep awkward conversations to a minimum. Besides, we were far too busy reliving our teenage glory days to fuss over flower arrangements.

After all, we had more pressing matters: namely, picking up exactly where we'd left off two and a half years before. Days on the beach, lazy lie-ins, laughing ourselves stupid over nothing. Any trace of cold feet or wedding jitters evaporated the moment we remembered we were better at fun than at being sensible adults. It felt absolutely right – the sort of perfect you only get when you squint really hard and ignore all signs of incoming doom.

Then – plot twist – we got married, and overnight Rebecca's mother and older sister decided they'd rather see me trampled by a stampede of kangaroos than accept me as part of the family. To this day, I have no clue what cardinal sin I committed. Did I breathe too loud? Chew incorrectly? Fail to read their minds and fulfil their secret fantasy of me spontaneously combusting?

Rebecca noticed, of course, but her reaction was gloriously underwhelming:

"They'll get over it," she said, with all the conviction of someone who'd clearly never met her own family.

Spoiler: they absolutely did not.

No matter what I did – whether I made a cup of tea, hung out the washing, or dared to exist in their vicinity – I was doing it wrong. And they, naturally, knew a far better way. They were the human equivalent of a 'one-star review' on TripAdvisor, only louder and living too close for my liking.

It didn't take long for the constant sniping to start leaking into our once-happy marriage like a slow, miserable gas leak. Arguments cropped up over nothing – but the real argument was always there in the background, in the shape of her mother and sister's rolling commentary on my general uselessness. I'm convinced they knew exactly what they were doing. They were subtle as a brick but twice as effective.

Eighteen months of this joyful domestic arrangement was about all I could handle. Somewhere along the way, all the laughing and lazy days got replaced by the sound of doors closing a little too hard. Eventually, we called it quits – not because we wanted to, but because my sanity politely said it couldn't handle any more.

Rebecca moved out.

We made a half-hearted effort to patch things up. We even went on a couple of "maybe it's not over?" dates. We were perfectly civil – a polite nod to our former selves – but the old spark had completely vanished. Maybe her mother had smothered it with a pillow while we slept. Either way, I stopped pushing it. I figured if Rebecca wanted to try again, she'd pick up the phone. She didn't.

In the end, the next time I heard from her was when a

fat brown envelope arrived through my letterbox: divorce papers, citing that timeless classic – "apart for two years, no chance of reconciliation." No dramatic phone calls, no war over who got to keep the bed linen. I signed the forms that very day and popped them back in the post.

And just like that, I was free again – older, slightly wiser, and with a brand new vow: if I ever get married again, I'm interviewing the in-laws first. Preferably with a lie detector and a restraining order ready to go.

Zena's Prophetic Words

Zena: "Look out for a girl with a man's name."

Mining is the biggest industry in Western Australia – a cheery fact which means beneath all that red dirt lurks every element the modern world can't function without. Iron ore, gold, copper, lithium, rare minerals which power your smartphone.

Naturally, these hidden treasures aren't found on the local high street but in blistering remote outposts where the summer sun turns your skin to crackling faster than you can say, *"Is SPF 50 enough?"* Entire camps – scratch that, mini-towns – have sprung up for the pleasure of housing these heat-baked FIFO (Fly-In-Fly-Out) workers.

Why do they do it? Mind-bendingly huge pay packets. In exchange for frying alive and missing your family for two weeks at a time, you earn enough to buy said family a new car every year – assuming they haven't forgotten who you are by the time you crawl back for your precious seven days of 'rest and relaxation.' Then it's rinse, repeat, retire with a bad back.

So, what did any of this have to do with me, the proud non-miner? Well, the mining gold rush vacuumed up half of Perth's able-bodied blokes and shipped them off to the desert, leaving the city embarrassingly short on people who knew one end of a hammer from the other. Enter me: Handy Andy – suddenly in demand, and more than happy to fill the handyman void for a decent wad of cash.

And what did I do with all this newfound wealth? Sensibly invest it? Save for my future? Don't be daft. The rent got paid – obviously, no one wants to be a well-paid hobo – then I fed myself like a king at the local supermarket, and KFC, and Maccas, and Hungry Jacks (Burger King to anyone outside Australia). Whatever survived the rent and food purchases found its spiritual home in the till at my new local watering hole: The Grand Boulevard Tavern, or GBT if you were part of the furniture like I rapidly became.

The GBT was a cavernous pub plonked in the heart of Joondalup – just a quick fifteen-minute wobble from the house Rebecca and I had rented shortly before she decided life with me was about as relaxing as a wasp in a bottle. Perth, being the show-off it is, has 300 days of sunshine a year, so naturally the GBT's shady beer garden became my new headquarters.

Now, I should mention I was still a 'dirty smoker' at this point – so spending my evenings perched under a parasol, chain-smoking and nursing pints of ice-cold Tooheys Extra Dry (Teds, to us seasoned boozers) felt like a pretty solid lifestyle plan.

Each evening, I'd gently insert myself into the pub's social fabric – a fabric woven from Aussies, Brits, Scots, Kiwis, South Africans, Irish and a healthy splash of god-knows-where. It was like the United Nations, except everyone agreed on one thing: the English Premier League was sacred.

It didn't matter if you hailed from Manchester or Mumbai – if you supported a Premier League team, you had an instant passport to pub citizenship. Russell, the GBT's ever-smiling owner, made sure every match was plastered across giant screens dotted around the place.

Sure, I had Foxtel at home – but come on, watching football alone on your sofa is basically shouting at furniture. Far better to stand shoulder to shoulder with equally deluded fans, shouting at each other *and* the telly. If a match fell within licensing hours, I was at the GBT. If it didn't, I begrudgingly moped back home and yelled at my own TV.

Now, you'd think being a Manchester United fan in an expat-heavy Aussie pub would guarantee me safety in numbers. Ha! Not at the GBT. Man United fans were a rare breed – an endangered species overshadowed by a Chelsea mafia who, naturally, took enormous pleasure in my misery any time United stumbled. And did they let me hear about it? Of course they did.

But football karma is a glorious thing – every time Chelsea slipped up, I made sure to be as gracious as a winning lottery ticket. They gave as good as they got; no hard feelings, just world-class banter and the occasional shouted profanity when the ref made questionable choices. Good times, good beer, good people – all lubricated by a river of Teds and self-delusion that *next season was ours.*

On Friday nights, us regulars would show up like clockwork at around 5.30 pm to enjoy a few pints and a lot of football debates. We rocked up earlier than normal because the GBT underwent a population explosion at 8 pm sharp, when an army of fresh-faced weekend warriors swarmed in like locusts who had just turned legal.

Anyway, back to Zena – my ever-mystical personal fortune teller. Remember her prophetic mutterings?

165

Well, one Friday night at the GBT became the living proof that she might've known more than I might have given her credit for.

One particular Friday night, I decided to make a grand entrance by turning up late. Not fashionably late – just late enough to guarantee I'd be publicly shamed for it. Sometime just after six, I barrelled through the GBT gate, slid into the bar like a man possessed, grabbed a pint of Teds, and sprinted to the beer garden where the regular Friday mob was already judging me with the warmth of an open freezer door.

My tardiness, naturally, had not gone unnoticed. Oh no. Within seconds I was dragged before a full-blown Kangaroo Court, starring the entire smug Chelsea contingent as judge, jury, and executioner. I tried the classic excuse: *"Sorry lads, got held up by a customer."* They heard: *"Blah blah excuses."* Verdict: Guilty. Sentence: One full round for everyone – which promptly murdered my bank account and left my wallet crying for its mum.

Once the pints were safely parked in front of the mob and the atmosphere had thawed slightly, I slumped next to Colin – a Fulham fan, bless him, proof that not everyone aims high in life. Beside him sat a young woman I didn't recognise.

"This is Charlie," Colin announced, with all the fanfare of a royal herald.

Charlie? That was a man's name. Mmm....

"Hello," I said politely. She echoed it back just as politely. And that was that – or so I thought.

166

Charlie was a Kiwi fresh off the South Island sheep paddock, and pretty soon she was clocking more GBT hours than the bar staff. Like me, she seemed surgically attached to her pint and her cigarette, but there was one tiny wrinkle: she clearly couldn't stand me.

Every night she showed up, she managed to sit as far away from me as possible without physically leaving the postcode. If I arrived first and claimed a prime beer garden table, I'd watch her do a full tactical sweep: come through the gate, spot me, do a silent *ugh,* grab her Jim Beam, and plonk herself at a table three diplomatic zones away. Subtle? Not remotely. Effective? Absolutely.

This went on for weeks. I was genuinely puzzled. I'd only ever spoken three words to her – *"Hello," "Hello," and probably "Cheers."* What mortal sin had I committed to earn this stealthy Cold War?

Then came an unexpected plot twist. One Saturday, having nobly decided I deserved a weekend off from DIY drudgery, I went shopping around lunchtime for things I didn't need. Naturally, this detour led me right past the GBT. And naturally, instead of continuing home like a normal person, I did the only logical thing: I went in. It was broad daylight, mind you. I rarely drank before 5 p.m. But it was five o'clock somewhere – that ancient rule of the semi-functioning alcoholic.

Armed with an icy pint and my cancer sticks, I staked out my usual beer garden throne and settled in for an afternoon of people-watching. Perth sunshine, cold beer, other people's conversations to eavesdrop on – life was pretty bloody perfect.

About ten minutes into my covert anthropology session, out came Eloise, her partner Bobby, and – surprise surprise – Charlie, trailing behind like someone facing a dental appointment. The garden was heaving, so naturally the only empty chairs in sight were at my table. Eloise, seeing this as divine providence, led them straight to me. Charlie looked like she'd rather share a seat with a nest of funnel-web spiders.

For the next hour, we all laughed, drank, and – astonishingly – Charlie didn't hiss at me once. You'd think we were best mates the way she joined in the banter. I still couldn't figure it out. What had changed? Did she mistake me for someone else? Did I have a halo over my head I wasn't aware of? I didn't dare ruin the vibe by asking.

A few hours and a power nap later, I was back at the GBT, now properly geared up for a Saturday night session. More Teds, same seat in the beer garden – living the dream.

Then who comes through the gate? Yep. Charlie. She spotted me, smiled (I swear!), and headed inside. I actually checked behind me to see if Jesus himself was sitting there and he had been the recipient of her friendly gesture. Nope – she'd definitely smiled at me. Maybe it was just trapped wind?

Moments later, out she came, Jim Beam in hand, but instead of her usual evasive manoeuvres, she strolled right over and sat next to me – voluntarily. At this point, I began to suspect I'd slipped into a parallel dimension.

We chatted. We laughed. Other regulars drifted in and

out, but Charlie and I were locked in a steady stream of conversation which carried us through the night. All that passive-aggressive avoidance? Gone.

Did I ask her there and then what my crime had been? Of course not – I wasn't about to jinx my new favourite drinking buddy. Some weeks later, curiosity got the better of me and I asked what I'd done to offend her delicate Kiwi sensibilities. She didn't miss a beat:

"I just thought you were an arrogant prick."

Well, fair enough. She wasn't wrong – but still, a bit harsh after a single hello. Then again, she was far from the first to reach that conclusion.

Cheers, Charlie. Fair play.

Man Utd 3 - Chelsea 1

Charlie and I had become the kind of pub regulars landlords dream about – reliably keeping their lights on and their tills overflowing, six nights a week and twice on Sundays if there was football on. And I, for one, was thrilled that Charlie's initial belief that I was an arrogant twat had faded into the warm haze of beer-soaked amnesia.

Despite spending half our lives together at the GBT, Charlie was still a bit quiet in the way cats are quiet right before they ruin your favourite sofa. Her sense of humour, though – that came through loud and clear, usually at my expense.

As you may have worked out, I adore Manchester United with all the pathetic blind faith of a true fan. Charlie, on the other hand, worshipped the All Blacks with the kind of obsessive patriotism only a Kiwi can muster – but had never, ever watched a single game of what she called "proper football". Not one. Despite the fact that, at the GBT, you couldn't sneeze without hitting a 60-inch plasma screen showing the Premier League.

One memorable Saturday not long after she started speaking to me, United were playing West Ham at Old Trafford, kickoff at the gentlemanly hour of midnight Perth time. The plan was simple: leave the GBT before closing, stumble home, and watch the inevitable United victory in my living room, undisturbed.

Purely out of politeness – and fully expecting to be rejected – I invited Charlie to join me. After all, she was young, fun, and surely heading off to Dusk, the local nightclub where everyone under thirty went to get completely pissed and make poor life choices.

At 11:30, she vanished inside the bar and reappeared moments later brandishing a six-pack like a warrior queen.

"Ready when you are," she declared.

What?! Apparently, I'd just bagged a personal cheerleader for the night.

On the walk back to mine, we demolished a couple of kebabs like two feral raccoons. Between mouthfuls, I confidently explained to Charlie how United were about to teach West Ham the meaning of pain and humility, because obviously Sir Alex Ferguson was the second coming of Christ and Old Trafford was basically football Valhalla.

Ninety minutes later, we'd lost 2-0 and my new apprentice football fan was politely trying not to laugh into her beer. It was character-building, alright.

In the weeks which followed, Charlie and I fell into a comfortable routine: we were pub soulmates. Same table, same round, same sarcastic banter. There'd be others at our table, but our little side chats were just for us. She was the highlight of my day – which probably says more about my day than I'd like to admit.

When I first met Charlie, she was crashing at her aunt and uncle's place. This ended about five minutes after they realised she enjoyed a pint too much and didn't clock in at bedtime like a Victorian orphan. So she upgraded to her cousin's house. My place was slap bang in the middle of her new digs and the GBT, so she started popping by on her way to the pub.

My work kept me busy – well, busy-ish. When I was focused, time flew. But when I knew Charlie would be knocking around 7pm, I spent the afternoon looking at the clock, wishing the hours would bugger off quicker so we could get to the important bit: beer, football arguments, and my quest to find out about all things NZ.

Right on cue, my doorbell would ring. We'd head out together like some middle-aged dad and his sarcastic adopted Kiwi daughter – only with more swearing (on my part) and cigarettes. The GBT staff quickly cottoned on: if you saw one of us, the other was probably loitering nearby.

Sometimes, of course, one of us would fly solo. Charlie occasionally ditched me for girly nights out – presumably to complain about my tragic fashion sense – and I sometimes rocked up late if I'd been trapped in a customer meeting listening to someone drone on about renovation budgets I had no intention of sticking to.

If I showed up alone, the bar staff would do the same interrogation routine:

"Where's Charlie?"

Me: *"How should I know? I'm not her bloody babysitter."*

Pint poured. Interrogation over. I suspect she got the same third-degree when she arrived solo. If she had a witty comeback, she kept it under wraps.

The rest of the GBT crowd were great drinking buddies but absolutely useless for anything beyond that.

Charlie and I were the only pair who did "real life" together outside the pub: random walks, humiliating bowling sessions (I say humiliating because she wiped the floor with me). She was twenty-five years younger than me, so any delusions of romance were parked firmly in the "don't be a creepy old man" zone. She was my mate. End of.

One night in 2008, I strolled into the GBT on my own and, before you even ask – YES, the staff demanded to know where Charlie was. I gave them the usual: *"I'm not her keeper, mate."* But secretly, I did know – she was in the city with another friend, screaming herself hoarse at a Foo Fighters gig while I was doing the important work of defending Manchester United's honour in enemy territory: surrounded by a gaggle of smug Chelsea fans.

That night was the big one: Chelsea versus United at Stamford Bridge. I was outnumbered at least ten to one, we were playing away, but I was ready for battle. The pub was buzzing – right up until the inconvenient reality that the GBT closes halfway through the match hit us. So, just before kickoff, the entire army of pub-based hooligans scarpered home to watch the carnage on our own tellies.

Final score? United 3 – Chelsea 1. I went to bed smugger than a cat in a sunbeam, ready to milk it for all it was worth the next time I saw the Chelsea lot.

Just as I was drifting off into a blissful sleep, my phone buzzed. A text. From Charlie.

Charlie: Are you still up?
Me: Why?
Charlie: Want to talk to you about something.

Me: Door's open.

You're Kidding, Right?

Was the door locked when Charlie texted me her midnight decree? Yes. So being the gallant gent I am (and more afraid of her than of any burglar), I dragged myself out of my warm bed, stomped downstairs, unlocked it like a tired concierge, then crawled straight back under the duvet, fully expecting to never hear about it again.

I drifted off at once. Peace at last – for all of twenty minutes.

Next thing I knew, there she was: Charlie. Laid on the bed next to me, gently shaking my shoulder, and staring at me like a Victorian ghost about to deliver my doom. If you've never woken up to a silent Kiwi's fixed stare, consider your blood pressure blessed.

Feeling unnerved – and deeply aware of my mortality – I broke the silence first.

"Well?" I mumbled, trying to sound braver than I felt.

Suddenly, she switched on like a lightbulb. Apparently, I was no longer single. According to Her Royal Highness Charlie, we were now *in a relationship*. Non-negotiable. I asked her to spell out exactly what that meant – partly because I couldn't quite believe I was awake, and partly because I hoped I'd misheard.

"You're going to be my boyfriend," she said, slowly and clearly, as if addressing a confused Labrador. "And I'm going to be your girlfriend."

I did what any sensible, cornered man would do:

"Yeah, right." And I rolled over and went back to

sleep, convinced the universe would reset itself by dawn.

When I next cracked open an eye, daylight was creeping around the blinds and I realised I wasn't alone in bed. I turned my head – and there she was. Charlie. Same deadpan stare, zero smile, full psychological warfare.

Fantastic. It wasn't a dream after all.

"So... remind me again. What was all that last night?" I asked, with the smug confidence of a man about to watch her backtrack and blame the Jim Beams.

I couldn't tell if she had been drunk the night before. I suspected she had been for her to say what she said. I was going to enjoy her embarrassment as she admitted to making a fool of herself. Yes, she had best-mate status at that point, but one thing we could do was laugh with each other and at each other. You couldn't! If you ever tried, we'd beat you to death. But between us, it was allowed.

Except she didn't backtrack. She calmly repeated it, word for word. Not a flicker of embarrassment. No second thoughts.

She was serious. Bloody hell!

So, naturally, I pulled out my Best Objections:

– The age gap!

– The inevitable day she'd wake up, realise I looked every minute of my years, and bolt screaming into the arms of a hot surfing instructor called Chad.

– Basic sanity.

Charlie demolished every excuse without breaking a sweat. Once she'd made up her mind, I could have hired a whole team of hostage negotiators and it wouldn't have mattered. Charlie wanted it, so it was happening.

In the end, I gave up – and made breakfast to celebrate my surrender. Priorities, right?

Over the next few weeks, I made several valiant – and utterly doomed – attempts to break up with her. Not because I didn't like her (I liked her far more than I was emotionally equipped to handle) but because the logical part of my brain knew this would end in me trying to keep up while she ran off with someone who didn't need a lie-down after three pints.

She ignored every attempt. She just kept showing up, more adorable and infuriating than ever, until eventually even my excuses packed up and moved out.

Very soon after, she moved into my townhouse – which basically involved her dumping a bag of clothes next to mine, claiming half the bathroom shelf space, and declaring one of the living room sofas her personal kingdom.

Now instead of just being pub buddies, we became that annoying couple who sometimes stayed in, ordered takeaway, and spent all night talking nonsense about everything and nothing. We still hit the GBT a couple of times a week to keep up appearances, but most nights we were at home, watching movies, mocking bad TV, and steadily building a fortress of inside jokes.

And yes – I became the biggest sap in Perth. If she finished work early, so did I. If she walked through the front door at 3pm, I pretended I'd just *happened* to knock off early too. Subtle? Not at all. Happy? Hell yes.

Obviously, it wasn't all candlelight and rainbows. We argued – usually about stupid things like who ate the last Tim Tam or whether my jokes were actually funny (they are). But there was one argument, a spectacularly ugly one, fuelled by the poisonous whisperings of a so-called friend who probably thought blowing up our happiness would make her own sad life feel less bleak.

And it worked. The fight got so out of hand that Charlie packed her bags and vanished back to her cousin's spare room – and decided I was persona non grata. Calls? Ignored. Texts? Read and ghosted. Showing up at her cousin's place? Oh hell no – Matt already thought I was an ageing creep corrupting his innocent relative. Knocking on his door was about as smart as poking a bear with a pointy stick.

So, I did what any lovesick fool does: went to the GBT every night like a stray dog waiting for its owner to come back. Everyone knew. Nobody asked. The bar staff just poured my beer in pitying silence.

One night, on a heaving Friday, I spotted her at the bar. My heart jumped. I pushed through bodies like a drunk salmon heading upstream – but by the time I got there, she'd Houdini'd out the back door like the world's fastest ninja. That stung more than I'll ever admit.

The townhouse seemed empty. All the furniture was as it was before, nothing visually had changed other than there being a lack of Charlie. Those lonely moments made me realise she hadn't just become a huge part of my life, she was my life. How had she managed to do that? The answer was simple. I was totally and utterly in love with her.

As you know, the only other girl I have ever loved, and still do, is NJP. When that came to a head, I reacted very badly and let her slip through my fingers. To this day I know I should have tried harder to win NJP's love. Here I was being given a second chance at love, I was not going to give in so easily.

So I did the only thing I could think of: wrote her a letter. An actual bleeding-heart email – no jokes, no sarcasm, just the truth about how that old witch had lied, how my life felt like a sitcom with no laugh track since she'd left, and how the only happy ending I wanted was the one with her in it.

I hit send. Then prayed she'd read it. Because if she didn't – well, the old trout who caused all this drama? She'd never get what she wanted anyway. Not even if Hell itself froze solid and started selling ski passes.

Please Come Home

A few days later, the doorbell rang. Charlie – who still had a perfectly good key, mind you – decided ringing the bell would add to the drama. When I swung the door open and found her standing there, I felt two things simultaneously: sheer elation... and raw terror. Whatever was about to happen needed to go exactly right. No room for my usual spectacular ability to put my foot in it.

For days I'd rehearsed what I'd say if this moment ever came. Hourly monologues, full Shakespearean soliloquies in the bathroom mirror. And now, with Charlie right there in front of me, every clever word promptly evaporated out of my head. So, naturally, like the brilliant strategist I am, I blurted out nothing useful, and somehow, in the middle of all that awkward tension, we agreed to go for a drive.

The car had always been our mobile confessional. On countless afternoons when we had nothing better to do, we'd just pick a random direction – North? East? South? – and let the wheels and our conversation wander wherever they pleased. No destination required. It was cheap therapy, and it worked.

This time, I didn't bother asking her which way she fancied. I pointed the bonnet south, pressed the accelerator, and prayed I wouldn't say anything stupid enough to wreck my second chance before we'd even hit the freeway.

I did my best to keep my voice casual, tossing out questions while trying to hide the fact I was internally sweating buckets. Charlie's replies were short, polite... about as warm as an accountant reading parking fines. But hey – she was talking, just. Which was better than door slams and radio silence.

About ninety minutes later, we rolled up at Falcon Beach, out past Mandurah. The sky was absurdly perfect – that smug, cloudless blue which makes everything look cinematic. The waves lapped the sand obligingly. And, best of all, the entire beach was ours.

We strolled along it slowly, no hand-holding, just two people doing their best impression of being casual strangers – except I couldn't help noticing she'd straightened her hair. And not just *straightened*, but magazine-advert straight. She knew exactly how good it looked. Was that her silent peace offering? Or a silent "Feast your eyes, loser – look what you lost"? Either way, guilty as charged.

An hour passed like that: one foot in front of the other, conversation stuck in first gear. When we reached a shallow pool left by the retreating tide, we naturally drifted to opposite sides. Ten metres apart, but it felt like miles. I watched her: hair catching the sun, wearing that pale blue sweater and old jeans, looking like everything I'd ever wanted and didn't deserve. In that moment, one blinding fact slammed into me: being without her would ruin me. Full stop.

Then it got weirdly vivid – the breeze, the seagulls, the sound of the waves sharpened, like life wanted to make damn sure I'd remember this snapshot forever. And oh, I do.

Eventually, she turned back towards the car. I fell in beside her, trying not to trip over my own heart. As soon as we crossed back over that puddle, closing the gap between us, I reached for her hand – almost bracing for her to pull away. She didn't. She didn't even flinch. Her fingers slid into mine like they belonged there. And that was that. We were back on track.

To this day, when I replay that afternoon, I can see it all: the exact shade of the sky, the salt in the breeze, the way she looked at me without looking at me. One of those rare memories which wraps you up in total happiness. May it never fade.

Charlie moved back in that very day. That night, because routine is comforting and beer is better than therapy, we walked up to the GBT. As we strolled through the gate, I spotted Lyndon and Janet – a couple of our usual partners-in-crime. Janet elbowed Lyndon and gave a subtle chin-flick in our direction.

Their faces lit up with huge grins – apparently delighted that Charlie and I had stopped being idiots long enough to sort ourselves out. Or maybe they were just relieved they didn't have to pick sides at the bar anymore.

Either way, they were pleased. But not half as pleased as me. I had my girl back – and with her, the map for my future snapped back into focus.

Hailstones and Other Madness

At some point during one of our many deep and meaningful conversations – probably sandwiched between sorting the laundry and scraping last night's dinner off the plates – I casually mentioned to Charlie that I'd love to drive around the entire country someday. You know, just one of those harmless daydreams people say to sound interesting, then promptly forget about once the washing machine beeps.

Not Charlie. Oh, no. She never forgets. While I wandered off to daydream about other impractical nonsense, she quietly adopted this particular fantasy as a personal mission. She didn't nag or pester. Instead, she sneakily built an entire 'Round Australia' dossier behind my back – pinning down destinations, researching must-see sights, probably planning which remote towns she could abandon me in if I got too annoying.

Then, one evening while we were both multitasking (I think I was heroically drying dishes while she loaded the washing machine), she casually asked,

"So, IF we ever did this... which way would we go?"

Easy. *"North,"* I said, like I'd given it deep strategic thought when, in reality, 'north' just sounded more adventurous than 'left'.

She nodded. Didn't say a word for weeks. Next time she did? Out came a master plan so detailed it looked like it had been drafted by NASA. Apparently, my passing fancy was now the official future, and Charlie was its CEO.

One evening at the GBT, seated in our beloved beer garden – our temple of bad ideas – we were mapping out how this escapade could possibly work. Enter J.J., our mate, local lunatic and self-declared philosopher, who'd done his own grand circuit back in the mid-seventies. His retelling, naturally, included heroic amounts of cheap wine, suspicious cigarettes, and near-fatal mechanical failures. It was pure comedic gold. We laughed so hard we nearly choked on our Tooheys. And all his misadventures only made our crazy dream sound even better.

A few days later, thanks to big-mouth J.J., our 'secret plan' was GBT gossip fodder number one:

"You two really driving around Oz?"

And before we could even answer, everyone piled on with their 'essential' recommendations:

"Mate, you gotta see Kakadu!"
"Broome, trust me!"
"Don't skip the Nullarbor – it's boring, but you have to do it!"

Oh, and J.J. insisted on Darwin. Why? Because he'd just scored a new job there as a Power Station Operator. He'd never actually been there on his own trip, but now it was top of the list because – surprise! – if he bought a fixer-upper, guess who'd be legally bound to renovate it for free rent and a carton of beers? Handy bloody Andy, that's who.

By October, our 'one day, maybe' idea morphed into 'yeah, we're actually doing this'. I even started warning my customers: *"Sorry, you'll have to find another sucker to unblock your toilet in 2010 – we're off!"*

And that's when the panic set in. Word spread faster than the flu in a kindergarten. Suddenly my phone exploded with calls which all started the same way:

"Before you go, can you just…"

And out came the shopping list of everything they'd ever wanted done since Federation.

Could I have just shut up shop and left them all high and dry? Technically, yes. But these people had fed Charlie and me – literally. Their leaky taps paid for our rent, our groceries, and the countless rounds we'd shouted at the GBT. I couldn't ghost them. So out came my trusty notebook. I personally visited every single loyal customer, handed them a pen, and said,

"Write it ALL down. Tonight. No extra 'while you're here's tomorrow. This is it."

Charlie, bless her restless heart, took the news like a champ. Our grand New Year's Day escape morphed into "sometime in June, maybe July, depending how many cracked tiles Mrs. O'Reilly finds behind her washing machine."

Had we stuck to our original plan, we'd have hit the road in our old Holden Commodore Station Wagon – the same noble beast I'd used to haul my handyman junk. Not exactly the Batmobile, but it would've done the job.

Fate, however, had a better plan: in April 2010, we scored a 'new' 4x4. Well… new-ish. Just before we bought it, a freak hailstorm pummelled every car yard on Scarborough Beach Road with hailstones the size of tennis balls. I kid you not, it looked like God Himself had gone bowling. The car yards, naturally, did what car yards do best: stuck giant 'DISCOUNT!!!' signs on everything with dents and hoped desperate suckers would bite.

Enter: us. Our 'new' 4x4 came with a free roof massage, a custom dimpled bonnet, and a few bonus cracks – but it also came with a seven-year drivetrain warranty. So if the engine spontaneously combusted halfway across the Outback, someone else would pick up the tab. Win. Charlie, still on her learner's permit, loved it – her first car, and it looked like it had just about survived an asteroid belt.

Next, we scored a second-hand trailer. Naturally, we over-thought it: we built a box on top, imagining we'd be smuggling priceless heirlooms through monsoons and desert cyclones. Spoiler: more than 75% of what we so meticulously packed turned out to be utterly pointless. Australian campsites have everything. We could have fit what we actually needed into a sturdy backpack – but no, we dragged that boxy monstrosity halfway round the continent.

And the tent – oh, the tent. That glorious 'necessity' stayed untouched in its pristine packaging right up until the day before departure. When I finally cracked it open to test-run it, chaos ensued: poles flew, pegs bent, curses echoed throughout the suburb. Charlie still cackles at the memory. She is proofreading this book before going to publishing and right at this point in the text, I'm betting she's doubled up crying tears of laughter at the memory.

But hey – we did it. Or at least, we were finally,

definitely, absolutely *about to*. Our grand Aussie road trip was real, our old handyman debts were settled, our battered 4x4 was primed, and our trailer was pointlessly stuffed with everything we didn't need.

Next stop: the wild blue yonder – armed with a questionable tent, far too many spare pillows, and enough stubborn optimism to conquer whatever hilarity the Outback would throw at us next.

The Road To Nowhere

Finally, on the 7th of July, 2010 – after what felt like a century of "Can you just...?" jobs – we rolled out of Joondalup at about 9am, pointed the car vaguely north along Indian Ocean Drive, and drove straight into our 'great Aussie adventure' with all the confidence of two toddlers with a map drawn in crayon.

Sure, the weather was miserable (because winter in Western Australia is nature's way of reminding you it does, in fact, have seasons), but the sense of freedom was unreal. Freedom with a spicy side of low-level dread: we had no clue what we were doing, and the Australian wilderness is the sort of place that can kill you with either a snake bite or existential boredom – dealer's choice.

Credit where it's due: Charlie had poured hours into plotting this trip. Almost every 'point of interest' she'd flagged kept us snuggled close to the coast. Our rhythm was simple: on driving days, we rumbled along for four or five hours, windows down, wondering if the trailer would survive the next pothole. On non-driving days, we lazed on deserted beaches, blasting our favourite music, or lay around our tent like contented possums. But every evening, without fail, we'd grab a couple of cold beers, plonk ourselves on a rock, a dune, or straight onto the sand, and watch the sun melt into the Indian Ocean. We never got sick of that bit – nature's free Netflix.

Jurien Bay, Horrocks, Port Gregory, Kalbarri, Denham, Exmouth – we drifted through them like backpacker ghosts. We never booked ahead, never planned how long we'd stay. Sometimes we packed up after one night. Sometimes five. The tent came down when we felt like it, and not a minute before.

Meanwhile, despite spending every waking second together, I genuinely started to forget what Charlie's actual face looked like – because it was permanently hidden behind her brand-new Canon camera. Three hundred photos a day? Bare minimum. To be fair, she was annoyingly good at it – genuinely professional stuff, no Photoshop required. I've often thought about printing them into a fancy coffee-table book, but there's just so many that picking which ones to include would cause a mental breakdown. So they sit on a hard drive instead, gathering digital dust.

Eventually, we pulled into Broome and stayed about ten days. Turns out Broome is so popular, it practically demands a booking six months in advance – which, naturally, we hadn't done. We circled every caravan park in a steadily growing panic until we found the absolute last available patch of dirt at a spot called The Pistol Club. No idea why it was called that, but I'd find out soon enough.

The place was run by another Charlie and his wife, Anna. In the off-season, it was just the two of them; in peak season – which, lucky us, we'd definitely hit – they drafted in help: Sheffield and his wife. Sheffield was a pleasant enough Pom, but also a terrifying hybrid of hall monitor and MI5 surveillance drone. He clocked my accent the second I said "Hello" and christened me "Bolton" for our entire stay. So naturally, I called him

"Sheffield" in retaliation.

Sheffield ran that campsite like the Ministry of Fun Police. Speeding around the site? Bollocked. Talking too loud after dark? Bollocked. Existing in a way he found questionable? Gentle bollocking. And weirdly, despite Charlie being at my side for every infraction, she never once got scolded. Everybody loves Charlie. Andy? Not so much.

My first run-in with Sheffield's iron fist approach came on our first Saturday night. We'd hit the Roebuck Hotel's Corona Bar for the afternoon (five bucks a bottle – it would've been criminal NOT to), cycled back slightly sideways, and then, genius that I am, I dragged out the Wii and a screen from the trailer to challenge half the campsite to a raucous round of digital golf.

More beers flowed, volume rose, dignity plummeted – until Sheffield materialised out of the shadows like an angry ghost. The crowd vanished in record time, leaving me stammering an apology while Sheffield explained, politely but firmly, that if I didn't shut up, I'd be evicted faster than I could say "birdie".

Then he turned, smiled sweetly at Charlie, and said, "Good night, Charlie," as if she'd spent the evening doing charity work instead of egging me on.

Twat!

Anyway, I staggered to bed, passed out cold, and was jolted awake hours later by what sounded like artillery fire:

CRACK!

I jumped Bolt upright.

"What the f### was that?" I hissed at Charlie, while wrestling with a ball of clothes I'd drunkenly dumped at my feet. Why I asked her – who was inside the tent with me – I'll never know.

Her eyes drifted shut again.

CRACK! Again. Closer. Louder. I was ready to crawl under the inflatable mattress.

"It's the Pistol Club," she mumbled. And it clicked: right, Pistol Club. It was literally a gun range. And apparently, the die-hard marksmen of Broome think 7am on a Sunday is a fine time to empty a magazine at some targets parked five metres from my fragile hangover.

As I flopped back onto my pillow, contemplating my life choices, I couldn't help but reflect on the irony: I'd nearly been evicted for a bit of Wii golf and giggling – but 9mm semi-automatic fire at dawn? Totally fine.

But hey, they had guns. I had a tent. So, fair play.

Once again, the open road gave us a seductive wink and beckoned us onward – this time, for the next level of 'What Could Possibly Go Wrong': a gentle 660-kilometre jolt along the legendary Gibb River Road, deep in the untamed wilds of the Kimberley region in Western Australia.

Let's clear this up for the uninitiated: when I say 'road', what I actually mean is 'a violently corrugated strip of compacted red dirt' masquerading as a highway. There's no soothing bitumen here – just endless bone-rattling ridges formed by torrential rains, bouncing you around like you're inside a paint mixer. Attempt it in a family sedan and you'll be airlifted out with your exhaust pipe embedded in your spleen. The Gibb River Road is for vehicles built like tanks, and drivers just reckless enough to trust their tank won't explode halfway through.

Fortunately for us, we had both: our battle-scarred hail-dimpled 4x4 and our unwavering faith that 'it'll be fine'. And so we rumbled on, rewarded at every punishing kilometre by scenery so stunning it could reduce even the most cynical soul to misty-eyed silence. Gorges which made you believe the dinosaurs might still be hiding in them; waterfalls straight out of glossy travel magazines – except better, because they weren't clogged with tourists wielding selfie sticks.

Honestly, if I had the vocabulary to do the Kimberley justice, I'd be selling millions of books instead of hammering this one out while drinking instant coffee. It really is one of Earth's last untouched Edens – a place that wedges itself into your chest and refuses to leave, long after your spine has forgiven you for the drive.

When we finally rolled into Kununurra, red dust in every bodily crevice and a suspension system whimpering for mercy, we felt a genuine wave of triumph. We'd done it. One of Australia's most notorious drives: conquered. Rattled within an inch of our sanity, but conquered. If there's a more beautiful wilderness out there, then the universe is just showing off.

Kununurra has precisely one caravan park (or so it felt to us), so we crawled in and claimed our patch of dirt. Charlie immediately announced she was starving and swanned off to hunt down dinner, leaving me – once again – to do battle with the tent solo. Now, you'd think after the twentieth time, a man might have mastered the art of tent erection. You'd be wrong. (Your laughing hysterically again, aren't you Charlie?)

Five minutes in, I was in full meltdown mode: poles jabbing me in the shin, canvas mocking me from a tangled heap, hammer launched dramatically in the general direction of the grass – narrowly missing our already pockmarked windscreen. And there, leaning against the 4x4, was Charlie, doubled over, wheezing with laughter like she'd bought front-row seats to a one-man circus called 'Watch Andy Lose His Shit'.

Eventually, pity overtook her amusement, and she stepped in to restore calm before I dented the car any further. Miraculously, we got the tent upright without involving paramedics.

After another blissful night beneath the Southern Hemisphere's glittering sky – which is gorgeous but does nothing to cushion a rock-hard ground – we packed up our rolling circus once more, waved goodbye to Western Australia, and crossed into the wild, ever-shifting scenery of the Northern Territory.

Next stop: more adventures, more bruises, and absolutely no sensible decisions in sight. Just the way we liked it.

The Northern Territory

A few days later, after surviving the Gibb River Road with most of our teeth still in place, we rumbled triumphantly into Darwin – the Top End, crocodile country, and, more importantly, home to our dear mate J.J.

We met him, naturally, at his local watering hole: The Beachfront Hotel. This fine establishment was in Rapid Creek, right across the road from his freshly purchased apartment – because walking more than thirty steps for a beer has always been against J.J.s religion.

By then, Charlie and I were so used to living under canvas that an actual roof, four walls, and a toilet which flushed felt suspiciously decadent. But J.J. insisted: "Stay as long as you want – rent free!" Of course, this is J.J., so 'free' came with strings. Specifically, a brand-new kitchen. He paid for the cupboards, sink and oven; I paid with my sweat, my patience, and my lower back. Fair's fair, I suppose – just don't ask how many beers were needed to keep me from fitting that oven upside down.

Darwin life quickly settled into a groove. Within a couple of weeks, I scored a sweet gig installing Venetian and roller blinds for a small company called Straitline Blinds – genuinely one of the best jobs I've ever had. Twelve people, zero drama, and all of them just decent humans who made work feel like an excuse for a good laugh. My off-sider, Zelio, and I zipped around town in the work van, transforming windows and pretending we knew what we were doing. If Charlie and I had decided to plant roots up there, I'd probably still be hanging blinds with Zelio today, gossiping about everyone else's crooked curtains.

Meanwhile, Charlie landed a housekeeping job at the Free Spirit Resort, just outside Darwin – fancy name for a caravan park with delusions of grandeur. She took the 4x4, I had my van, and life in the Top End was pretty sweet.

By March 2011, I'd finished J.J.'s dream kitchen (with only minor swearing and no major plumbing disasters). But apartment life – and J.J.'s 'eccentricities' – were starting to gnaw at Charlie's sanity. She wanted back on the road. Who could blame her? So, we stuffed our worldly possessions back into the trailer, turned the car south, and hit the Stuart Highway towards Tennant Creek like a pair of dusty nomads who'd overstayed their welcome.

Leaving Darwin, the sky was postcard-perfect – brilliant blue, not a hint of doom. The temperature hovered in the thirties, the soundtrack was upbeat, and our optimism was sky-high. Naturally, the universe saw this and thought, Not so fast.

Within an hour, that glorious Top End weather turned into a monsoon of biblical proportions. What started as 'refreshing drizzle' escalated to 'holy crap, are we driving underwater?' in record time. We slowed to a crawl, wipers on warp speed, eyes straining through a windscreen which might as well have been made of frosted glass.

Somewhere halfway down the NT, we swung east onto

the Barkly Highway – aiming for Mt. Isa in Queensland before nightfall. Ha! Nightfall? We'd have been lucky to have made it by Christmas at the rate we were progressing.

Every patch of sketchy phone reception brought another text from Kevin B, my ex-colleague at Straitline. Kevin, bless his meddling soul, was tracking the weather – and us – with unnerving accuracy. I started wondering if he'd duct-taped an AirTag to our trailer. His updates were helpful though:

"Storm cell ahead – good luck, mate!"

"Next 50km: solid rain – keep crawling!"

Gee, thanks, Kev.

Meanwhile, the Barkly turned into a single-lane slip-and-slide. We couldn't pull off the road because the verges were now soup. Getting bogged in the middle of nowhere in an Australian wet season is a special kind of stupid, so we stayed on the tarmac, creeping forward whenever we could see more than a metre ahead.

The worst fear wasn't so much hydroplaning into oblivion – it was a 60-metre road train ploughing up our backside while we sat there like stunned mullets. Every time we stopped, I half-expected to see headlights looming behind us, followed by our 4x4 being turned into a pancake.

It was twelve hours of white-knuckled terror, our soundtrack a mix of AC/DC (ironic, given the circumstances) and the sound of our wipers sobbing in protest. When we finally limped into Mt. Isa, alive but traumatised, I realised something: AC/DC's Highway to

Hell must have been written right there on the Barkly Highway, mid-downpour, with a soggy map and an empty petrol tank. Nothing else explains it.

But hey – we'd survived another chapter of 'Andy and Charlie's Excellent Misadventure'. Queensland, you'd better be ready for us.

And it was. I thought the last twenty four hours had been a nightmare. That was nothing compared to what Mt. Isa had in store for us.

Trailer Trashed

Dead on our feet and wired on pure survival instinct, we finally rolled into Mt. Isa just as the sun – hidden behind an apocalyptic blanket of rainclouds – threatened to rise in the east. The rain still poured, though now with the gentle subtlety of a brick through a window rather than the full Noah's Ark re-enactment we'd endured on the Barkly.

We hadn't eaten in eighteen hours, our nerves were frayed like a two-dollar phone charger, and if we didn't get food soon, one of us was bound to gnaw off a limb. Lucky for us, Mt. Isa's main street offered plenty of vacant parking spots – because no sane human was out sightseeing in this Godforsaken monsoon.

I swung out of the driver's seat on legs that barely remembered how to stand, shot a suspicious glance at our battered trailer and wondered: How much of our worldly crap is now soup? But honestly, opening it up to find out would have required emotional strength I did not possess.

And right at that specific moment, because the universe clearly wasn't done mocking us yet, the trailer decided to quit life altogether. The wheel bearing on the driver's side disintegrated in spectacular fashion. In one miserable clunk, the wheel cocked itself forty-five degrees, the axle folded like a drunk uncle at a wedding, and the whole trailer slumped over as if it'd just been kneed in the family jewels.

"F###!" was the only appropriate reaction.

We stared. It leaned. The rain poured. I seriously considered setting the whole thing on fire and claiming alien abduction on the insurance form.

But Charlie, saintly and infuriatingly calm, reminded me we needed breakfast first – because obviously, collapsing trailers can wait but an empty stomach cannot. And as always, she was right. So we trudged off through soggy Mt. Isa in search of coffee and greasy food, leaving our poor, wheel-maimed trailer to sulk by the curb.

Charlie's biggest superpower? Optimism. Even with bacon and eggs finally taking the edge off my murderous rage, I was ranting about how the trailer could have picked ANY OTHER TIME to drop dead. She just shrugged and called it "part of the adventure." Is it any wonder I'm hopelessly in love with this infuriatingly positive woman?

Back at the scene of the crime, the trailer – shockingly – had not healed itself in our absence. A thorough inspection confirmed my worst fear: it was well and truly f#####. Beyond the help of a hammer, duct tape, or gentle pleading.

So now what? Unhitch the whole sorry mess, abandon it on the street, and continue our epic odyssey with nothing but a boot full of wet socks and regret? Tempting.

But once again, Charlie's brain kicked in before mine did. "Why don't we just go find a replacement?" she chirped, as if new trailers grew on trees in Mt. Isa.

Spoiler: they do not. We slogged through torrential

rain, poked our heads into every dodgy yard and sad industrial lot in town, and turned up exactly zero second-hand trailers. If you ever wondered where trailers go to die, it's apparently not Mt. Isa.

What Mt. Isa did have was a shiny new trailer yard – the only one within a million kilometres. They knew it too, the smug bastards. Negotiating for a cash discount? Hah! Price on the tag, mate. Take it or leave it and good luck towing your busted heap back to Perth.

Two grand lighter and still soaking wet, we then faced the next level of Mt. Isa hell: the Queensland Licensing Department. The bloke behind the counter had obviously had a charisma by-pass but did have a very irritating pen-clicking habit which made my eye twitch.

Apparently, buying a trailer was the easy bit. Registering it and getting a registration plate required me to have a Queensland driver's licence.

My license was a Western Australian License, which bore my Joondalup address where I no longer lived. In an ideal world, which I was about to find out Mt. Isa was definitely not part of, I could have transferred my WA license to an address of a friend, but that could only be done at a Western Australian Driving Licensing Centre. But we were in bloody Queensland! Try explaining nomadic homelessness to a pen-clicking desk jockey with the imagination of a boiled potato.

It quickly escalated to a full-scale bureaucratic nightmare. I needed a Queensland address to get a Queensland licence to register a Queensland trailer. But we didn't have an address because, newsflash, WE LIVED

IN A CAR! The concept of us being travellers, which by definition meant we didn't currently have a permanent address, seemed to blow his tiny mind.

At the precise moment my blood pressure hit critical, Charlie stepped in and charmed Captain Clicky Pen into revealing we could use a hotel address. So back out we went, stumbling through puddles and ginormous potholes and generally getting pissed on, in search of a single vacant room.

We eventually found a gin-soaked motel owner who slurred something about "room seven" and after dropping the key more than once, waved us vaguely towards it. I'd have hugged him if I didn't think he'd collapse. We paid for a single night because we'd sooner sleep in a crocodile-infested swamp than stay in Mt. Isa a second longer than necessary. As soon as we had that god forsaken plate, we we're out of there.

Armed with our shiny fake 'residence', we returned to the licensing dungeon. An hour and forty new forms later, I had a Queensland licence which looked like it had been typed and laminated by a five-year-old who had never used a laminator or a typewriter in their short existence on the planet. So unprofessional was the finished product, if someone had presented it to me as ID when I was running pubs and clubs, I would have laughed at them and showed them the door. But apparently it was valid, so whatever.

Next step: the trailer registration. A slightly more functional human behind the counter accepted our mountain of paperwork and announced we could collect the rego plate the next morning providing the paperwork was all in order.

Morning? I wanted to scream. But Charlie dragged me outside before I could throw myself through a window.

She reminded me we had a motel bed paid for, and she was determined to squeeze at least one perk out of this soggy hellhole. Fine. I didn't want dinner – I wanted booze. LOTS.

She flipped through the local 'what to do in Mt. Isa' leaflets and decided we were going to The Buffs – a club promising cheap beer, hearty food, and entertainment which would hopefully go some way to distracting me from my rage.

So we showered, suited up in raincoats, and trudged off through Mt. Isa's swampy streets in search of redemption. Miraculously, The Buffs delivered: cold beers half the price we were used to, food so good I nearly wept, and live music which helped me forget my deep, seething hatred for bureaucracy.

If you ever find yourself trapped in Mt. Isa and you can't get out before sundown, do yourself a favour: hit The Buffs. It might just save your sanity. As for the rest of Mt. Isa? I hope a sinkhole opens up and swallows it whole.

Rain, Rain, and More Bloody Rain

Shockingly – and I do mean shockingly – the following morning everything actually went to plan. I half-expected the new trailer to spontaneously combust or the registration lady to change her mind overnight, but no. Within the first hour of business, we had the shiny new rego plate bolted on, the old trailer left abandoned on the verge for the trailer place to dispose of, and we were rolling east once more through the never-ending biblical downpour.

Next checkpoint: Townsville, that scenic patch on the map where rain goes to retire. From there, the cunning plan was to swing a left and head straight up to Cairns – except Mother Nature and the Department of Road Closures had other ideas. Seems entire chunks of highway had been washed away in the storms, and trees along the route were teetering at gravity's mercy, ready to squash unsuspecting road-trippers like us.

No one had a clue when this 'minor inconvenience' would be fixed – maybe tomorrow, maybe next century – so, in the spirit of spontaneous detours, we shrugged, cursed, and hung a right southward to Airlie Beach instead. If you can't drive north, you might as well find somewhere with bars and cheap beer, right?

Airlie Beach did not disappoint. We drowned our frustrations with a full-blown bar crawl which lasted a suspicious number of days. Between hangovers, we caught up on the local gossip, which included the glorious news that the highway north had reopened – at least as far as Ingham. Before anyone could slam the boom gates shut again, we frantically packed up our living equipment and made a break for it.

At Ingham, we stopped roadside to inhale greasy burgers while the electronic signs told us the road was 'closed'. As we stood there willing the electronic sign to change its mind, we witnessed an entire convoy of trucks rumbling out from the supposedly impassable route. Clearly, they knew something the sign didn't. Next second, the lights flicked from angry red to come-hither green, and I had us back on the bitumen before Charlie even finished chewing.

Sure, it was still raining – obviously – but the wipers on speed one could finally keep up. Five soggy hours later, we rolled into Cairns... and miracle of miracles, the sky suddenly decided it had tortured us enough and turned off the tap. Not a single drop fell the entire time we stayed. Cheers for that, Weather Gods.

Accommodation? Well, the first three nights we 'camped' in the car, which was romantic for exactly seven minutes before it turned into cramped, sweaty hell. Luck eventually threw us a bone in the form of a ground-floor apartment rental – the entire bottom half of a house, no less. The landlords, Colin and Chris, lived upstairs and, thank the beer gods, loved a party. For three months straight, every half-baked excuse was good enough for a knees-up, and naturally, we were always on the guest list.

Now, just before we graced Cairns with our presence, Cyclone Yasi – the worst tropical hissy-fit Queensland had seen in living memory – had obliterated large

204

chunks of the region. Hotels, businesses, tours – smashed to bits. So while we sipped beers at Colin and Chris's impromptu shindigs, we did wonder if maybe our being there was a tiny bit tactless. Us trying to get employment where employment was scarce, we were just adding to the problem.

Our bank balance was circling the drain faster than our leftover beers. There was money gushing out but a suspicious lack of money trickling back in. So, naturally, each day we set off to 'job hunt' with the best of intentions – only to be ambushed by the Courthouse.

Now, you'd think a courthouse would mean official business. Not this one. This courthouse had been repurposed in the best way possible: as a pub. And every single day we 'just happened' to drift in for 'just one'. Which always turned into four – because they sold Coronas for $3.50 a bottle, and we were powerless in the face of such reckless generosity. Did we ever leave sober? Take a wild guess.

In between all this productive beer research, I landed a short stint fixing crash-mangled caravans – good fun, but over in a blink. I also did a few gigs fitting blinds for an interior designer whose 'steady stream of work' turned out to be more of an occasional dribble.

Charlie, meanwhile, threw her hat in the ring for a job running a car rental agency. There were five thousand applications for just one position and she made it to the final two. Any sane person would have high-fived themselves for beating 4,998 people – but not my Charlie. She was furious about losing to that one smug sod who actually had experience running a car rental place. Outrageous, right?

And so, with no steady work and no clear future, the writing was on the tropical wall: time to hit the road. Had things been different, maybe we'd still be perched on Colin and Chris's porch, beer in hand, spinning yarns about how we survived Yasi's aftermath. But, as Australia's favourite bushranger, Ned Kelly, once said: Such is life.

Bye Bye Cairns, Hello WA

It was a Sunday afternoon at the end of June when we gave Colin and Chris a final round of hugs, heartfelt thank yous, and swore blind we'd keep in touch (we didn't). We'd been on the road for days shy of a year – for the most part living wildly, spending freely, and pretending we were carefree drifters instead of two functional adults eventually doomed to rejoin the workforce. So, with hearts heavy and a bank balance lighter than helium, we did the sensible thing and headed back to where we knew we could flog ourselves for a paycheque: Western Australia.

We rattled south through Queensland, zig-zagged New South Wales, crossed South Australia, endured the mind-melting tedium of the Nullarbor, and rolled back into Perth around five in the afternoon, six days after setting off. Pretty efficient, considering we didn't lose a wheel bearing or a trailer this time.

Monday morning, no messing about – resumes in hand, hair combed (ish), we hit every hospitality mob which serviced remote mine sites. Because when you're broke and marginally employable, nothing says 'smart life choices' like FIFO. Within the week, the tactic worked: we were both gainfully employed – on different sites, for different companies naturally, because the universe loves a good practical joke.

Firmly ensconced in the FIFO circus, we started casual: same swings, same R & R (Rest and Relaxation) blissfully synchronised. Home, for R & R periods, was a modest three-bedroom rental in Clarkson, a nondescript suburb about 15 Kms north of Joondalup where we'd lived before gallivanting around Australia pretending to be nomadic backpackers.

Our new routine? Two weeks of mining-site mayhem, one glorious week off to pretend we were normal people again. It was the longest we'd ever been apart since the day we met, so naturally, we did the clingy-couple thing and called each other every night. Our respective 'handlers' at work even bent over backwards to keep our rosters aligned – proof that miracles do happen.

And then, naturally, it all went to shit.

Without warning, my handler vanished on 'extended leave' (I suspect they snapped and ran off to Bali). Her replacement – let's call her Ms. Clueless – seemed to think synchronised rosters were a quaint suggestion, not an ironclad necessity to keep relationships intact. She started offering me every conceivable combination except the one which matched Charlie's: three weeks on, one day off, then ten days on, four days off – basically guaranteeing I'd see Charlie sometime after Christmas if I was lucky. It was September.

Being 'casual' meant I could reject jobs. And reject I did – with gusto. But after a while, living off fresh air and optimism wasn't exactly sustainable.

Meanwhile, Charlie's company, operating on a similarly dubious recruitment policy, at least had the sense to recognise a loyal workhorse when they saw one. We pleaded our case: hire me too, pretty please. They said yes – but with a catch the size of the Great Sandy

Desert: they needed me on a juicy megabucks construction project. Four weeks on, one measly week off. Quick mental maths confirmed we'd both be home at the same time once every nine weeks. Somebody wasn't understanding the problem we were trying to overcome.

I wasn't about to sign up unless Charlie was guaranteed a slot on the same site. Easy fix, right? No! And it was Charlie who was the issue.

Charlie's problem, and therefore mine, is that she puts her heart and soul into whatever she does. She is the kind of employee no site wants to lose. The manager where she was based flatly refused to let her go. He demanded the company replace her with someone with equal ability and willingness to work before he would even contemplate releasing her.

After much negotiation, we eventually came away with the promise that Charlie would be on the same site as me within three months. It was better than nothing. Nothing would have seen me looking for another job rather than taking the obscenely lucrative offer being put before me. Of course, once Charlie was on the same site, she too was going to be earning the same huge money I was being offered.

So we endured nine glorious weeks apart – romantic, huh? – but true to their word, exactly three months later, Charlie rocked up on Barrow Island and all was right in our FIFO world. For the next three years, we toiled like draft horses, shovelling our paycheques into the bank while sacrificing our sanity. Twenty-eight days on site, half a day either side wasted on travel, leaving precisely six days at home to unpack, repack, and briefly remember where we lived.

Meanwhile, smarter companies on the island cottoned on that the rosters being endured for 12 hour a day shifts were inhumane and shifted staff to rosters like twenty-seven days on, ten days off. Our lot? Nope. They were determined to milk every last drop of blood, sweat, and tears from us. But hey – we'd signed up for it, so no right to whinge.

By November 2013, Charlie decided we were sufficiently cashed up and politely informed me it was my call when to jump ship. She was itching to escape back to a cushy production gig with a civilised roster (2 weeks on, 1 week off). Lucky her – her wish came true the following July.

One morning, I got into an almighty barney with a supervisor – and won, technically. When I was interviewed after the fracas, Management backed me up, told me I was right. They asked me to withdraw my resignation which I handed in verbally during the argument. Within the hour of the initial set to, Charlie, working in a different department, heard about what happened and also tendered her resignation. To be fair, management did their best to get us to reverse our decision, but we both knew it was time to call time on the most well paid gig either of us had ever had. Of course, we did agree to finish our final 28 day swing because we are clearly masochists.

My daily routine hadn't changed during my time on Barrow: up at 4 am, inspect the bus I'd spend my shift driving around in, breakfast in the dry mess, then my caffeine ritual in the wet mess while absorbing whatever drivel the ABC called 'News'. In all that time, the Project Assistant Manager never once graced the wet mess at 4.30 in the morning. But the minute our resignations hit her desk, guess who started dropping by daily to chirp, "Good morning, Andy! Changed your mind yet?"

Lady, for the zillionth time – NO! And yet she persisted, right up to the day we waved goodbye to Barrow Island from window seats on the plane.

Old Blighty

Within a couple of weeks of once again being spectacularly, heroically unemployed, we booked ourselves onto a plane bound for the UK. Now, if the holiday destination argument had ended with me being victorious – which, let's be honest, it never does – then that wide-bodied jet lifting off from Perth International would have been soaring blissfully south-east, bound for either Auckland or Queenstown in New Zealand, where I'd planned to spend at least a month pretending to be a rugged adventurer while nursing a pint by a log fire.

But alas, 'She Who Must Be Obeyed', also known as Charlie, decided it was high time she met the brave souls who'd been forced to raise me, and to see for herself the mystical land where my questionable personality was forged. So the UK it was. Democracy at its finest.

In all fairness, and with gritted teeth, I must admit: it was bloody brilliant. Charlie was an overnight sensation. My mother pulled her aside every spare minute to interrogate her about how she'd managed to transform her shambling son into a semi-functioning adult with acceptable table manners. My old man was genuinely puzzled, staring at her, then me, then back at her, trying to crack the Da Vinci Code of how I'd bagged a woman half my age and ten times classier. Our Kid, meanwhile, did her best to intercept the endless parental grilling to keep Charlie sane.

As for the rest of the family? They practically knighted her on the spot. Apparently, for my extended clan, having an actual New Zealander in their terraced house was the next best thing to a royal visit. She was paraded about like an exotic curiosity – "Look at her! She talks funny and everything!"

We did the full nostalgia circuit: The Lake District in Cumbria, a damp, wind-swept pitstop in Bolton where I first appeared on this earth, and a whimsical detour to Portmeirion in North Wales – the weird, pastel-coloured village where the '70s TV series *The Prisoner* was filmed. I even subjected her to the crime scene that was my old school, plus the Vic, plus a dozen more places which would bore the pants off any sane person – but she lapped it up.

However, there was one place she had burning a hole in her bucket list that I'd have happily skipped for the rest of my days: The nation's capital - London.

I'd done my tour of duty in London, thank you very much – interviews, boring corporate meetings, head-thumping rock concerts, nerve-wracking football games. Each time, I very quickly escaped The Smoke the instant my obligations ended, eyes watering from the diesel fumes and wallet traumatised by London prices. In my mind, London was just a giant, overpriced treadmill with bonus vagrants and pigeons on performance-enhancing drugs.

But Charlie had dreams. So, four days – *FOUR DAYS!!!* – in a Paddington hotel it was. I protested, naturally:

"Why not just an afternoon? Or better yet, a postcard?"

But Charlie brandished a to-do list which looked less like an itinerary and more like a screenplay for a ten-part epic.

We didn't stroll around London. We didn't even walk around London. We attacked it like caffeinated marathon runners. If we weren't hoofing it between attractions at breakneck speed, we were wedged on a big red open-top bus where I'd collapse exhausted while she ticked things off her manifesto.

But....and I hate to admit it... we had a glorious time. Every second of it. Somehow, and I've never managed to work out how she does this, but Charlie managed to make me see London through fresh, un-jaded eyes – like I was a tourist standing in front of Big Ben for the first time, instead of a grumbling expat with tube rage. If I ever do London again, I'd want her by my side, holding the map, ignoring my whining.

Soon enough, it was time to head to Wales, and my mood swerved all over the emotional highway during the drive down the M6 and the M5, and into the fairytale twisty roads of the Wye Valley.

Our first pit stop was Cardiff, where we landed in a pub with Dave, Tim, Tim's sister Augustine (always Augie to us), and her husband Phil. It had been a whopping sixteen years since we'd last laughed ourselves stupid together while pretending to sell exotic cars for a living. Two years working side by side had made us more siblings than colleagues, and falling back into that banter was like slipping on an old leather jacket which still smelled of beer and bad decisions. We didn't skip a beat. Charlie sat at the heart of it all, giggling at stories which painted a far less dignified portrait of her boyfriend than I had carefully crafted over wine at home.

Next on the nostalgia express was Bridgend – my old stomping ground, probably the place which had the biggest effect on shaping me into the semi-respectable reprobate I am today. As we parked at the small hotel, an uneasy knot formed in my gut. So much history there: friends made, enemies accidentally created, memories both cringe-worthy and glorious – and one unforgettable night still reigning supreme as the best of my life. Would bringing Charlie here blow the lid off things best left buried?

We dropped our bags, freshened up, and went exploring. Walking those streets was like flicking through a photo album you'd hidden in the attic: familiar places now ghosts of themselves. The Valbonne – the club which had been responsible for dragging me into town and spat me back out a changed man – had been demolished and was now a plain car park. But as we passed, I didn't see cars. My misting eyes saw the entrance lobby, the till by the door, the elevated bar in front of which I first hired NJP (and the same office where I spectacularly un-hired her later). I could almost see her storming out, her exit seared into my memory by a certain rear view which is still my final mental snapshot of that night.

As we wandered deeper into town, her memory trailed me like a ghost – was she still around? Still married? Had she moved on? I half expected her to pull up beside us at a traffic light, window down, same smirk.

I had floated a reunion invite on Facebook a week prior, hoping to lure old friends (and maybe old flames?) into one of our more familiar haunts for a pint or two and a laugh. Did she know about it? Had word been passed on to her? Would she come? Did she care? Did anyone?

That night, we detoured to Porthcawl for drinks with Martin and Teresa – faces I hadn't seen in more than two decades, not since Martin had swapped greasy overalls for an accountant's suit in Sheffield. Seeing them again was like seeing your reflection in a time warp: older, wiser, still game for mischief. Charlie soaked up every story about my misspent youth that Martin knew like she was researching for a scandalous biography.

The next day we drifted around Bridgend's streets and sights. I soaked up memories while discreetly scanning passing cars – as if NJP or maybe even Nikki T would magically appear behind the wheel. Nikki was another chapter altogether: drop-dead gorgeous, a laugh riot, and probably the only person (besides my mother) to have successfully steered my life onto a slightly less destructive path back in the 80s. She'll be making a grand entrance later in this book.

Evening rolled round and it was time for the big test: the reunion pint at The Three Horseshoes, the pub I spent time working in after my decision to quit The Valbonne. I braced myself for tumbleweeds – or worse, perhaps just me and Charlie nursing lonely pints while the current locals wondered who let the weird foreigners in.

Instead, the door swung open and bam – 1986 all over again. Same faces (a touch more 'character lines', a smidge less hair), same raucous laughter, same instant dive into a lot of stories best forgotten, but gleefully resurrected for Charlie's entertainment.

That night was liquid magic: hugs, roars of laughter, rivers of booze flowing like we were twenty somethings again and bulletproof. Old mates caught up, secrets spilled, Charlie grinned from ear to ear, immersed in my past lives which even I hadn't unpacked properly until then.

Between rounds, I slipped in a few quiet questions about NJP and Nikki T – no luck. They were ghosts tonight. Maybe just as well. Some stories need a little mystery to stay perfect.

And that, dear reader, is how you revisit the ghosts of your past, armed with a Kiwi, a camera, and a determination to prove that your best days might just still be ahead of you.

Back To Reality

Like all good things – ice cream, Friday nights, and my hairline – there comes a time when the fun must grind to a reluctant halt. The holiday came to an end. Charlie had the time of her life, and, to my utter shock, I found myself thoroughly enjoying what I'd originally written off as an ordeal to be endured rather than savoured.

Etihad Airways dutifully flapped us back to the so-called *Lucky Country*, where, as soon as the jet lag wore off, the awkward question of "What the hell are we going to do with our lives now?" began lurking around like a stray cat at a fish market.

First stop: check the bank balance. To our delight (and minor disbelief), we weren't destitute. There was no urgent need to paper the streets with résumés begging for someone – anyone – to hire us. So, we did the only sensible thing: we turned "funemployment" into an Olympic event.

We played golf. We continued attacking the half-finished renovations on the house we'd picked up in the sleepy coastal village of Two Rocks. We went on spontaneous road trips, disappeared for a few days at a time – and when we got home, we played even more golf.

Neither of us had any real golfing talent to speak of, but it gave me one rare thing: a sport in which I could routinely beat Charlie. So, whenever she trounced me on the PlayStation (we'd levelled up to a PS3 by then – yes, we're that old), I'd drag her out for eighteen holes of poorly executed revenge. It was a mutually agreed balancing act for our fragile egos. And so, in a routine of sand wedges and sandpaper, we managed to convince ourselves we were retired for more than eighteen months.

Retirement was good for me. It gave me the chance to cash in my "I choose the next holiday" card. In January 2016, we packed our bags and headed to a place I'd been daydreaming about for years: the fairy-tale land of New Zealand.

Now, I could bang on for pages – entire volumes, actually – about what NZ is all about. But no matter how many lyrical paragraphs I pen, I will never be able to do it justice. It's a place so breathtaking it makes the rest of the world look like it's not really trying.

It's a place which looks spectacular regardless of whatever the weather is doing. If you've never been, for the love of whatever deity you believe in, slap it on your bucket list *immediately*. You are categorically not allowed to die until you've driven its winding roads, gawped at its snow-capped peaks, and had a cup of tea with one of its outrageously lovely locals.

Why God hid this masterpiece in the farthest corner of the Pacific is beyond all comprehension. Maybe to keep it safe from people like us. And it worked – it's still unspoilt, jaw droppingly pretty, and inhabited by the friendliest folk you could ever hope to bump into.

At the beginning of my NZ enlightenment, we landed in Auckland, right up there in the north. We hired a car, and drove all the way down both North and South

Islands to Roxburgh where Charlie's family reside. It was a road trip I feel blessed to have experienced. New Zealand's stunning beauty, the warmth of the welcome from Charlie's family, the friendliness of the natives, all concluded with me boarding the homeward bound flight at Queenstown airport with a very heavy heart and almost in tears.

Back home in Two rocks and feeling as though I had left a huge part of me back in New Zealand, we had a *tête-à-tête* about what came next in our lives.

As any financially irresponsible adult will tell you, there's a limit to how long you can ignore the dwindling figures in your bank account before you have to crawl back into the workforce. After almost two years of living like rock stars on holiday, we realised the money pit had become more of a money puddle. The résumés were dusted off once more.

It was déjà vu all over again: same spiel, same interviews, same outcome – we ended up employed by different companies at different mine sites. But, thanks to Charlie's uncanny knack for persuasive negotiation (and a bit of harmless manipulation), I was soon dragged onto her site at Roy Hill Iron Ore mine.

For the first couple of years, we both worked for the hospitality company which ran the mining village – or as I liked to call it, *The Hilton in the Outback*. This place was less dusty work camp and more all-inclusive desert resort, with amenities which would make some city hotels look second-rate. It was a dream posting, if you didn't mind the odd snake, spider, and searing heat.

We both worked in Transport and Grounds: chauffeuring half-asleep miners to and from the pit, playing taxi driver to the airport, and moonlighting as amateur groundskeepers in between bus trips. We mowed lawns, fixed sprinklers, and pretended to know the difference between a weed and an ornamental shrub. It was bliss.

But then, the whisper of *bigger money* drifted through the bar during an after-work beer. We began making friends with the big shots in the Training Department. Soon enough, one of them leaned in conspiratorially and said, "You two should be driving trucks. Big trucks. The *real* money trucks."

Well, say no more. Within months, we'd wrangled our way into the operator's seat of Caterpillar 793Fs – giant yellow monsters the size of a respectable three-storey suburban house. At full load, each one weighed about five hundred tonnes, yet somehow felt like piloting a slightly oversized shopping trolley.

Once I'd mastered the basics, I discovered an unexpected problem: soul-crushing boredom. Twelve hours of crawling in circles, back and forth, with nothing but red dirt and your own thoughts for company. Meanwhile, Charlie was living her best life, dead-set on becoming Roy Hill's Queen of the Dump Trucks. And she absolutely would have done it too – I could see it within her first forty-eight hours in the cab.

In 2019, however, fate – and a careless lighting tower – conspired to cut my dump truck driving career short.

It was about three in the morning during a night shift.

Charlie and I were on the same roster, and we pulled our trucks into the same brightly lit Go Line for a break. We shut our trucks down and headed for the crib hut. As I strolled away from my truck, the generator powering the lighting gantry ran out of fuel and died an untimely death, plunging everything into pitch-black nothingness.

Being the graceful gazelle that I am, I didn't slow down. I tripped spectacularly over a pile of rocks which moments before I hadn't even noticed. I hit the ground with all the elegance of a falling wardrobe. It hurt like a punch in the ribs – probably because, as it turned out later, it *was* a punch in the ribs, courtesy of Mother Earth.

Stubborn as always, I got up, brushed off the pain, munched a sandwich with Charlie in the crib hut, and then climbed back into my truck for another four hours of back-and-forth torture. By the end of the shift, I celebrated my survival with a couple of beers – pain still humming under my ribs like a hidden alarm.

By evening, when I tried to get up for my next shift, I discovered I could barely roll out of bed without seeing stars. Somehow, I crawled to my supervisor, who decided I was a complete lunatic for not calling it in immediately. He marched me, slowly, to the On-Site Medic, who confirmed the obvious: ribs don't like being introduced to rocks at speed. I was benched, declared unfit for work, and pumped full of painkillers.

Drugged, bruised, and feeling like I'd been tackled by a bus, I endured the bumpy flight back to Perth for more poking and prodding. Final verdict? A nice clean rib fracture. No dump trucks for me for at least three months.

The End of an Era

Once I was back on my feet – ribs mostly intact and pride only moderately bruised – I knew I couldn't face boring myself into an early grave behind the wheel of a dump truck ever again. Call me dramatic, but twelve hours of trundling back and forth along the same five-kilometre stretch, serenaded by mind-numbing drivel being spouted on the two-way radio, is enough to turn anyone into a conspiracy theorist or a serial tea drinker. I had to find something else, preferably something which didn't involve crawling in endless circles at a pace which would make a tortoise yawn.

Of course, choosing sanity over soul-crushing repetition came at a price: more time apart from Charlie. By then, we'd clocked up about eleven years together, most of it spent blissfully stuck to each other like we'd been wrapped in duct tape. The impending reality meant we were about to become one of those FIFO couples – together in spirit, separated by a thousand kilometres of desert, and a roster which laughed in the face of romance.

In hindsight, I suspect that was the beginning of the end for us – not with fireworks or a screaming match, just a slow drift, like two dinghies untying themselves from the same jetty.

As the weeks ticked by, I threw myself back into my old handyman business – resurrected from the ashes like a very average, slightly under-qualified phoenix with a rusty toolbox. Whenever Charlie came home for her R &

R, I did my damnedest to clock off the hammer-and-nails gig so we could squeeze every minute out of our time together. But even then, something felt off – like we were play-acting the closeness we used to have, while living separate lives for two-thirds of the time.

I know she felt it too. But neither of us said it out loud. Some truths don't need subtitles.

In February 2020, she came home, sat me down, and said the words I half-knew were coming but still hoped were stuck in traffic somewhere on the Great Northern Highway: *what we had was over.*

To be honest, the reality of no longer being boyfriend and girlfriend didn't knock me sideways as much as losing my best friend did. And that's the bit that still catches in my throat, even now, four years on. Say what you will about soulmates, twin flames, or whatever spiritual mumbo jumbo people sell on Instagram these days – the truth is, she wasn't just my romantic partner, she was also my best mate.

After we split, I spent more time than I care to admit replaying our entire relationship like a cheap DVD stuck on loop. Should we have just stayed mates from the beginning? Should I have fought harder to stay on the same mine site, soul-crushing boredom be damned? But every time, my answer lands back where it started: *Absolutely not.*

The relationship I had with Charlie was the best I've ever had – and probably ever will have, unless Scarlett Johansson loses her mind and moves to Two Rocks. We had more than twelve years of adventure, idiocy, and enough inside jokes to fill a stand-up routine. If I could rewind the clock, I wouldn't change a single second.

Sometimes, when I'm feeling nostalgic (or when the Wi-Fi's down and Netflix won't load), I open up the digital treasure chest of the twenty-five thousand photos Charlie snapped during our time together. I scroll until my eyes glaze over, then close the folder with a grin which makes me look borderline deranged to anyone passing by my window.

Do I still love Charlie?

Hell. Yes!

A breakup doesn't magically dissolve love like sugar in tea – not for me, anyway. Just like my love for NJP – another glorious story involving a single unforgettable night nearly thirty-eight years ago which never went anywhere, yet still flickers away in some dusty corner of my brain whenever Rick Astley comes on the radio.

Truth be told, I count myself ridiculously lucky. I've fallen in love with two incredible women in my lifetime, which is two more than some poor sods ever get. If NJP had said "yes" instead of "no" that fateful night, I'd probably never have crossed paths with Charlie.   But meet Charlie I did, and what followed turned out to be the best twelve years of my life so far.

So Charlie was leaving, Covid was coming, and me? I was suddenly single in a world where toilet paper was about to become more precious than gold. But the curved ball lurking around the corner, I was not prepared for.

Health Problems

In November 2019, I finally admitted that the cough I'd heroically endured for a few *years* might just be more than a quaint little "smoker's cough". Charlie, bless her eternal patience, had been badgering me for what felt like forever to go and see a doctor.

"Go get it checked out," she'd bark, each time with an octave more frustration than the last.
Being the stubborn mule I am, I brushed her off every time. It'd sort itself out, wouldn't it? Maybe it was just my lungs clearing out decades of 'character building'.

Two years before this reluctant medical epiphany, I'd triumphantly ditched a forty-two-year smoking habit, only to leap enthusiastically into the warm embrace of vaping. I swapped the comforting stench of tobacco for delightful flavours like Coca-Cola and Strawberry Milkshake. If vaping had offered bacon flavour at that time, I'd probably have ordered a truckload.

During my time as a smoker, I used to say I *enjoyed* the taste of tobacco. That, dear reader, is utter bollocks. No one enjoys it. Smokers just grit their teeth until the brain is bullied into accepting the vile taste as normal. Don't believe me? Quit for five days, light one up, and watch your face contort like you just licked a tramp's armpit. Then, because we're all masochists at heart, we do it again until it's "normal" once more. Hooray for addiction!

So, armed with my new fruity flavours, I naïvely assumed my hacking cough would magically pack its bags and leave me in peace. God only knows where that logic came from – I suspect the same corner of my brain which believes leftover pizza is a balanced breakfast.

Predictably, the cough stuck around, unbothered by my wishful thinking, and Charlie's nagging only gained momentum. Some mornings were worse than others (I mean the coughing, not the nagging – although both could break Guinness World Records). Once I'd survived my daily lung eruption – anywhere between two minutes and a quarter of an hour of rib-bruising convulsions – I'd go about my day like nothing had happened. Perfectly normal, right?

Eventually, I cracked under Charlie's relentless badgering and booked an appointment with my GP. Brave, I know.

In his office, after my dramatic recount of near-death-by-coughing, he slapped his stethoscope on my chest, the metal freezing enough to make me squeal, and then asked me to "breathe normally". Sure, Doc. Let me just do that while my nipples are threatening to sue for frostbite.

He listened intently while he stared off into the abyss. Maybe he was daydreaming about his lunch. Suddenly he spun to his computer and tap-tap-tapped out a referral to a specialist at Sir Charles Gairdner Hospital, and handed it to me like he was giving away a free pen whilst assuring me, with a grin, that it was "precautionary". Well, if it was serious, surely he'd have said more. Right? Right.

Outside in the sunshine, I congratulated myself for paying $70 to be told I might not die just yet. Worth every penny.

At that time, the Aussie tabloids were frothing about our Medicare system being in meltdown: no beds, zombie doctors staggering through 72-hour shifts, equipment shortages, and patients abandoned to die in basement broom closets. Naturally, being a card-carrying member of the uninsured masses, I braced myself for a three-year wait and a hallway bed next to a leaky mop bucket.

But, lo and behold – within ten days, I was striding into Charlie Gairdner's (Aussies do love shortening everything). Either the newspapers were full of shit (never!) or I was closer to becoming best buds with the Grim Reaper than my GP dared to admit.

Inside, no patients were decomposing on trolleys. No panic. No doctors sprinting by screaming "Get me a crash cart, Stat!" like a bad episode of *Grey's Anatomy*. Everything was clean, calm, and suspiciously efficient. Damn the tabloids.

Before seeing the specialist, I was marched off for a round of "breathing tests", which turned out to be medieval torture disguised as modern medicine. Who would have thought repeatedly holding your breath for thirty seconds and then exhaling your soul through a tiny tube is a normal diagnostic procedure. Not me.

My tormentor – sorry, nurse – barked, "Keep pushing! Keep pushing!" with all the glee of a drill sergeant on meth. She might have been a descendant of Irma Grese (The Beast of Belsen - Google her if you dare).

After an hour of this aerobic punishment, I crawled,

gasping and traumatised, up the stairs to Dr K's office. My test results had digitally teleported far more quickly than me and were emblazoned across the screen of his laptop when I finally arrived and plonked my ass down in the seat he offered me. At least I think it was my results, it might have been an image of his 3 year old daughters finger painting.

Once I looked like I was revived, he hit me with the bombshell: "You have COPD."

"COP-what-now?" I asked, praying it was a cool new TV show.

Nope. It meant a charming cocktail of possible emphysema, asthma, and bronchiectasis.

Well, fantastic. My mind instantly flashed back to the late seventies when a mate's dad had emphysema. I was introduced to him in his kitchen where he sat at the table like Darth Vader's dying cousin – grey skin, blue lips, and a hissing oxygen tank which clicked as he breathed and looked like a prop from *Doctor Who*. Was that my future?

Sensing my panic, Dr K quickly back-pedalled: it *might* be mild, manageable, not full-blown "iron lung required" just yet. Still, he wanted me to quit vaping – apparently the jury was still out on whether it was better or worse than cigarettes. But either way, he wanted my lungs filled with good old-fashioned fresh air. Bloody spoilsport.

So, I left the good doctor's office mostly relieved but a tad rattled. That night, 27th November 2019, I went home, demolished two bottles of Shiraz, and vaped my brains out one last glorious time. Farewell, nicotine. We had a good run.

I haven't smoked or vaped since. Occasionally, muscle memory makes my hand grope for a phantom packet on the car seat, but I catch myself before the ghost ciggie hits my lips.

5 Months later, I was back for round two of the lung torture, and lucky me, Nurse Irma Grese was still on duty in the Chamber of Death.

Charlie tagged along this time, having magically appeared home from her FIFO gig. Dr K broke the good news: I'd smashed my breathing tests (take that, Iron Lungs Irma!) and the scary emphysema and bronchiectasis were off the table. Mild asthma was all that remained. I'd dodged a bullet yet again – I started to believe myself and Neo from *The Matrix* might have been one and the same.

Dr K gave me a puffer to use every morning, which basically stopped my daily phlegm spectaculars. Win.

As we had entered the Cardio unit prior to the breathing tests, we noticed a flurry of frantic activity outside the next building – people in Hazmat suits dashing about like actors in an international disaster movie. It reminded me of a Dustin Hoffman film I can't be bothered to Google. Dr K explained it was all prep for some new thing called Corona Virus. Apparently, I should avoid that too. Was this man on a personal mission to ban everything fun from my life?

We didn't bother explaining that Charlie was now mostly living four hours away with her new bloke – we just nodded and agreed she'd do the shopping and crowds bit. Best not complicate things.

So, off I went, free from vape clouds, armed with an inhaler, and determined to keep dodging life's bullets a little longer. Then Corona virus (Covid 19) crashed into the world, flipped everything upside down, and gave me one more reason to stay home with my Shiraz – sans vape.

Back At The Quacks

In late April 2020, I found myself perched once again in my GP's office. Why exactly? Who knows. Maybe for a flu jab, maybe for a repeat prescription for my daily puffer, maybe because I'm a hypochondriac in denial – take your pick. All I remember is that we were creeping into the soggy embrace of winter here in Western Australia and, apparently, I thought a doctor's waiting room was the place to be.

Just as I was about to lever myself out of the chair with all the grace of a retired rodeo bull, the doctor peered over his computer and asked, all casual-like, *"When was the last time you had your prostate checked?"*

I shot back, "You're the one with the computer, you tell me."

He clicked away with the enthusiasm of someone searching for cat memes, then announced it had been *"a while."* How long is *a while*? A week? A decade? I wisely kept that question inside my head and filed it alongside the other great mysteries like "Where are all my matching socks?" and "What exactly is quinoa?"

Since the nurse was still lurking about, he suggested I offer up some blood while I was there. One "small scratch" later, I was out the door, feeling rather smug about having ticked off yet another item on my "Pretend To Be A Responsible Adult" list.

A few days later, the surgery rang me. *Could I pop in to discuss the results?* Should I panic? Apparently not, according to the receptionist who chirped, *"Oh, it's just routine, duty of care, follow up, blah blah.*" She sounded so breezy I almost asked her for the next day's lottery numbers.

Fast forward to me, once again on my GP's paper-covered couch. He looked like he'd just stepped on a snail barefoot. My PSA level, he informed me, had come back *high*.

PSA. Three letters which mean absolutely nothing to most blokes – until they do. Even now, I couldn't tell you what PSA stands for (Prostate Something Something?), and honestly, I don't care. I just know the number that day was *12.6*, which, judging by his furrowed brow, was about as welcome as a fart in a lift.

Apparently, a high PSA can mean something sinister: *possible* prostate cancer. But, "*before we got ahead of ourselves*", he said, how about another blood test? Something about false positives – which, in doctor-speak, means *"We're going to make you sweat a bit longer, just for fun."*

While he siphoned more blood out of me like a vampire in scrubs, he attempted to soothe my spiralling thoughts by telling me how *slow* prostate cancer usually grows. He tried so hard to sound upbeat I almost felt sorry for him. Apparently, five of his other patients had been through it, and all were now fine and skipping through meadows cancer-free. He even mused that if he ever got cancer, *he'd hoped it would be prostate cancer*.

I resisted the urge to congratulate him on this deeply comforting fantasy.

To be fair, I'd heard this "slow cancer" spiel before

from an old Barrow Island workmate who'd been diagnosed a few years back. His doc told him that old age would kill him long before the cancer did – an oddly reassuring statement that now replayed in my brain like a bad TikTok loop. So, I shrugged it off and continued living life as if I didn't have a PSA level pushing double digits.

Three days later, my GP himself rang. Not his receptionist this time. *Him.* That's never a good sign. He'd cleared his calendar to squeeze me in *the very next day.* That little voice inside me (the sensible one I ignore most days) muttered, *This isn't going to be good news, champ.*

The new results were in: 12.6 had grown to 13.4 in just a few days. Even with my limited medical prowess – most of which comes from late-night Googling – I knew that was not good. No more talk about cancer being as harmless as a hangnail. He promptly referred me to a specialist. Things had officially become *serious*.

Once again, cue the much-maligned, supposedly 'broken' Medicare system. It still wasn't broken. It swooped in to help me like Batman. Within days, I was in a clinic, pants around my knees, lying on my side while a specialist rummaged around my rear end like she'd lost her car keys up there.

If you've never had a rectal exam, here's my advice for when you do: don't try to break the tension with a clever joke. You might think you're being hilarious – trust me, you're not. The doctor's finger is going to do what the finger must do, and the last thing he or she wants while exploring your darkest crevices is a stand-up routine.

Stay silent. Clench your dignity, not your buttocks, and don't make a twat of yourself.

When she finally removed her skeletal probing digit – and flung the glove into the biohazard bin like a grumpy magician – I asked, "So, what were you feeling for, exactly?"

She explained she'd been checking whether my prostate was enlarged, and if it felt hard, soft, or had the texture of badly laid concrete. Apparently, a lumpy, rock-hard prostate is bad news. Smooth and soft is better – though, unfortunately, her fingers were neither. And how did she know what badly laid concrete felt like? Were the cancer rates dropping to such a level that she needed to career change to a builder on the weekends, performing kitchen extensions and the like?

Next stop: a biopsy. She would do it herself at Joondalup Hospital – assuming she wasn't moonlighting as a bricky to pay off her student loans.

Again, the public system impressed me with its speed. Within two weeks, I was snug in a hospital gown, waiting to be sedated.

One thing I genuinely enjoy about hospitals? Anaesthesia. That delicious moment when they say, *"Count backwards from ten,"* and your brain says, *"Nah mate, I'm clocking out at seven."* And just like that – darkness. Blissful, dreamless darkness.

This time, I remembered reaching seven and hearing a bloke say, *"He's gone."* And I was.

Ten days later, the results of the biopsy were back in the capable, concrete-laying hands of my specialist. They didn't exactly deliver the triumphant all-clear I'd been daydreaming about. As she'd suspected, those pesky cancer tumours were indeed loitering in my prostate like unwelcome houseguests – but the biopsy was just stage one of figuring out the full horror show. Were the tumours politely staying put, or had they packed their bags and gone on a sightseeing trip through the rest of me?

If they were confined to the prostate, surgery was on the cards. Of course, "surgery" always sounds so neat and clean until you learn about the little bonus features, like the high risk of nerve damage. Nick that central nerve and you can wave a tearful goodbye to any future "good mornings" in the trouser department. I don't know many blokes keen to give that up – at my age, a bit of morning glory is a small but reassuring victory.

So far, I'd been poked up the bum, biopsied, sedated, and prodded within an inch of my dignity – yet I still clung to the vague belief that a quick treatment would sort it all out. Bit of an inconvenience, couple of pills, back to normal, right?

Wrong.

Before the oncologists could plot their next move, I needed a PET scan – basically a high-tech game of "Where's Wally?" but with cancer cells instead of stripy blokes. No drama there: I lay on a tray in a hospital gown, got shunted back and forth through a giant humming donut, and was home before lunch. No needles, no pain, no worries.

At that point, Charlie had moved into her new

boyfriend's house, and whilst she was still FIFO, when she was home, she lived a four hour drive away. Yet, she was still determined to support me. When I had appointments, she offered to fly home early from her Pilbara swing to accompany me – but I kept brushing her off. I was sure I had this handled, plus wasting her hard-earned leave days for what I still believed was a minor speed bump seemed daft. Cancer? Pfft.

My dream team consisted of two oncologists: Dr. W, the radiotherapy and hormone therapy wizard, and Dr. P, the chemotherapy connoisseur. Appointments with each were scheduled a week apart. Charlie, bless her FIFO soul, was on-shift for the first one but promised to come with me to see Dr. P the week after. At the time, I asked her mainly to be polite – turned out I was very glad she came.

When the day arrived for the meeting with the first Oncologist, I parked myself in a waiting area of Charlie Gairdner's, half-expecting the usual two hour wait. To my shock, Dr. W himself popped out right on the dot and called my name. I nearly checked my watch to make sure I hadn't slipped into an alternate universe.

Dr. W was one of those rare humans who instantly put me at ease – not just because he ran on schedule (though that did earn him serious points). He had a calm smile, a soft voice, and the gentle manner of a man who seems so accommodating he probably apologises to traffic when he walks over a zebra crossing. If I had to guess, I'd peg him at late thirties, maybe early forties – though given my track record at guessing ages, he could just as easily be twenty-five or pushing sixty.

He ushered me into his office, offered me the good chair, and spun his laptop around so I could see the technicolour horror show inside me. He scrolled through the PET scan images, giving a gentle running commentary like David Attenborough narrating a wildlife documentary – except the wildlife was neon yellow cancer spots.

Apparently, the tumours hadn't just set up camp in my prostate; they'd expanded the franchise into my lymph nodes too. The official term was "metastasised," which sounds very medical but basically means "your cancer's got a passport and likes to travel."

While gently dropping this bombshell, Dr. W did his best to balance it with the good news: cancer treatments have come a long way in the last fifteen years. While my brain processed phrases like "never going to go away" and "manage the problem," he calmly explained that his job – along with Dr. P's – was to slow this unwanted squatter down for as long as possible.

One tool in his kit was hormone therapy. A simple injection of a drug called Lucrin, once every three months. Its mission: put the cancer cells to bed and keep them snoring.

"So what happens when they wake up?" I asked, my optimism having taken a noticeable kicking.

"If or when they do, we have plenty more options in the arsenal," he said, still smiling reassuringly. Nothing to worry about then?

Up until that moment, I'd naïvely believed there were only two ways to fight cancer: chemotherapy and radiotherapy. Hormone therapy was news to me – and apparently, I could be on it for the rest of my days. Dr. W said it so matter-of-factly I almost felt guilty for not having a plan to live forever.

He walked me back to the waiting area himself – nice touch – and I thanked him for what he was about to put me through.

Strolling through the sunlit car park, I replayed everything he'd said. In short: one Lucrin jab every three months, plus chemo from Dr. P, and maybe radiotherapy later if my poor body hadn't had enough excitement by then.

When he'd finished laying out my options, my response was instant:

"Where do I sign?"

I didn't have private health insurance, but Medicare had my back like a dependable older sibling. Going with Dr. W's plan was a no-brainer.

Did I grasp how deep in the proverbial I really was? Probably not. Dr. W did his best to make it clear, but I suspect I didn't want to know – at least not yet. The penny, as they say, was still stubbornly clinging to the edge of the slot and not dropping.

One week later, on 23rd July 2020, I found myself in the nurses' area of my GP's practice, trousers lowered to mid-thigh level, and bum cheeks waving hello to the world like two pale balloons at a sad birthday party. Nurse Rochelle – who should honestly teach a masterclass in painless stabbing – deftly launched a needle into the juiciest part of my backside, pressed the

240

plunger, and sealed the crime scene with a single round band-aid. I didn't feel a thing as my first dose of Lucrin started its grand tour of my bloodstream. Night night, cancer cells – sweet dreams, you miserable squatters.

Charlie was with me, because of course she was – apparently four-hour drives and FIFO rosters don't stop her from playing chauffeur, therapist, and drill sergeant, all rolled into a 170 cm powerhouse. Our next port of call was Sir Charles Gairdner Hospital, to meet Oncologist Number Two: Dr. P, the Chemotherapy Guru.

We sat in Dr. P's waiting room. And sat. And sat. Dr. P's concept of punctuality was – let's just say – theoretical. Over the coming months I'd discover that not only was he incapable of being on time, he managed to be spectacularly late even for 9am slots, the first of the day.

Eventually, the door to his office swung open. Out shuffled a family moving like they'd just stepped off a battlefield – mother, father, two daughters – tears leaking freely, hands clutching shoulders and elbows and whatever was within reach. Even before Dr. P opened his mouth, I knew they were having a very bad day. Watching them stumble past us was like seeing my own future walk out the door: gut-wrenching, yet somehow I couldn't look away.

Then it was my turn to join the parade. Dr. P gave us a tight, funeral smile and waved us into the newly grief-cleansed office. He gestured to two chairs with the same warmth one might show a tax bill. We sat. He opened my file exhibiting all the ceremony of a man unwrapping a death certificate.

His voice – soft, syrupy, like he'd borrowed it from a children's television presenter who moonlights as an undertaker – dripped out of him in carefully rehearsed platitudes. But at least he didn't faff about. He went straight for the jugular.

"Your cancer is Stage Four."

Boom. Mic drop. Penny drop. Everything drop.
It was the first time I'd heard the words 'Stage Four' attached to my sorry carcass. And they landed like a sledgehammer right between my ears. All that cautious optimism I'd been carting around? Gone. Evicted. Vaporised.

He talked some more but I wasn't taking in what he was saying. The only thing I heard was me asking,

"How long have I got, Doc?" – because that's what every doomed protagonist says in the movies, right?

"At least two years," he cooed, lips curving into what might have passed for a smile if it hadn't been doing such a poor job of hiding the sadistic thrill of delivering bad news for a living.

Did I half-expect him to rub his hands together like a cartoon villain and cackle, *"Mwahaha!"*?

After that, whatever else he said might as well have been whale song. Words dribbled out of his mouth but all I heard was the pounding echo: *"At least two years... two years... tick tock, tick tock, tick tock..."*

I felt Charlie's hand on mine – an anchor in my private horror show – and I thank every available deity she was there, because without her, I'd have nodded, drooled, and probably signed up for chemo, snake oil, and maybe a free funeral plan all at once. She listened while my brain replayed my sudden expiry date on a miserable loop.

By the time we staggered out of Dr. P's office, I had apparently agreed to chemotherapy. Or maybe Charlie agreed on my behalf – who knows? I sure as hell wasn't operating heavy machinery in my mental state.

Like the devastated family before us, Charlie hooked her arm through mine as we shuffled back along the corridor, two newly minted members of the Terminal Club. To call her my rock is an insult to geology. She was a fortress – and I, quite frankly, was a damp paper bag with a hole in it.

Outside, the sun mocked me with its cheerful blaze across a cloudless blue sky. I pressed my back against a brick wall, I needed the support. I cried. Proper, ugly, snotty, can't-breathe sobs. Charlie stood beside me, clinging to my hand like she could squeeze the cancer out by sheer force of will. She cried too, though she'll tell you she didn't.

Eight weeks of vague horror had finally crystallised into one unshakable truth: I was going to die. Not 'someday' – but 'soon enough for a calendar to be insulting.' The medical plan was now crystal clear: delay the grim reaper, no guarantees, no promises of a sunset cruise into old age. Just a game of 'Let's See How Long We Can Stretch This Out Before the Lights Go Out.'

How much of that "two years" would I spend horizontal, high as a kite on morphine? How much would

I spend as me – the me who still cracked jokes and yelled at the TV? I didn't have an answer. Neither did Dr. P.

I don't remember how long we stayed pinned to that wall or how long the tears flowed, but eventually I scraped myself upright, lungs emptied of self-pity for at least a few minutes, and Charlie steered me toward the car.

I collapsed into the passenger seat like a rag doll. Charlie got behind the wheel. Neither of us moved. She stared at me, eyes red but defiant, waiting for my cue.

I stared through the windscreen, seeing everything and nothing. Dr. P's embalmed voice looped in my skull: *"At least two years..."*

Then, clarity. Rage. Stubbornness. Call it whatever you want – it flared bright enough to cauterise the fear.

I turned to Charlie and spat at the universe:

"Fuck cancer! I'll die when I'm bloody well ready to die! Not when some overpaid chemotherapist tells me. Let's go."

And with that, my war began in earnest.

Plans and Promises

It was late afternoon by the time we crept out of Perth's urban sprawl and pointed our little BMW north, up the Mitchell Freeway toward Two Rocks – our wind-battered, salt-sprayed corner of the world. The radio dribbled out forgettable pop songs, but neither of us gave it so much as half an ear. Charlie drove, eyes locked ahead, mind clearly somewhere far away. Mine? It swung back and forth like a rusty gate in a cyclone: *I'm doomed. Nope, I'm going to fight this. Nah, I'm screwed. Actually, no, I'll beat this, watch me.*

Charlie had decided she wasn't driving back to Dongara that night. Officially, the excuse was the four-hour drive through pitch-black bushland – a bad idea at the best of times, suicidal without a steel-grade roo bar and floodlights stolen off a mining truck. Unofficially, she just didn't trust me to be alone with my thoughts and a house full of sharp objects. Fair call.

Truth be told, I was relieved. There were about ten thousand things about my life I regretted at that point – but having Charlie next to me, even now that she lived with someone else, was never one of them. No one else would do for the kind of meltdown brewing within me.

If that night was going to be our last proper one together, I didn't want to waste it staring blankly at the telly or brooding over a sad takeaway dinner. And the local pub, full of nosy drunks who thought a tequila shot solved cancer, was off the table too. So, practical as ever, I asked her to swing by the bottle shop. If I was facing my

245

own mortality, I wanted a carton of beer in my corner.

I half-expected her to scold me about drinking myself stupid when I was already half-broken inside. But she didn't. Maybe she needed it as much as I did. Maybe the thought of me sober was even scarier.

Back at our battered beach shack – held together by memories, sweat equity, and enough silicone sealant to caulk a cruise ship – we settled at the tall table out the front. Across the road, the V-shaped dip in the dunes framed the Indian Ocean perfectly. That view had always been the house's best feature – the one thing we never had to mortgage or renovate.

We cracked open our first stubbies and watched the sun lower itself into the ocean like it had nowhere better to be. Dozens of sunsets had come and gone over that horizon – but tonight, it felt different. More final.

For twelve years, Charlie had been my sounding board, my moral compass, and my unofficial crisis manager. If I was going to come up with a plan to attempt to keep myself alive a little longer, I couldn't imagine doing it with anyone else.

So we got to work. Or, more accurately, she did. I mostly drank and nodded a lot and let my thoughts bounce rapidly between negative and positive.

If you've read my history in the first part of this book, then you know I didn't exactly treat my body like a temple. More like a testing ground for everything the human liver can (and shouldn't) survive. Beer? Practically a food group. Cigarettes? A loyal friend until recently. Food? If it came battered, deep-fried, or wedged in a cardboard box, I was your man. Exercise? Ha! If you count sprinting away from the cops once or twice in my youth – then sure, I was an athlete. Otherwise, I avoided sweating like it was an allergic reaction.

So maybe I'd earned my diagnosis. But knowing I'd invited cancer in didn't mean I was planning to let it kill the host without a fight.

According to Charlie, because I zoned out real fast after Dr.P's first couple of sentences, his grim revelations had left me with two choices: endure months of medical battering which *might* buy me time, or do nothing and coast on "at least two years" – part of which would probably be spent drooling into a pillow in a hospice bed. Neither option was exactly an Ibiza holiday package.

He had informed us the treatments open to me would be exhaustive. Charlie deciphered his words to mean I was going to have to be mentally, physically and emotionally ready for what was to come.

Was I ready? Not even close.

It was time for honesty. I had to face up to the truth. I was a physical, mental and emotional train-wreck.

I could change that but first, I needed to answer one serious question. Did I want to live, or did I want to die?

Sitting there with Charlie, with the sunset doing its best impression of a Hallmark postcard, I knew one thing for certain: I wanted to live. I wanted every scrap of time I could squeeze out, preferably with some dignity left and maybe the odd sarcastic quip. I wanted time to fix everything I'd ruined for sixty-plus years.

Over the years, I had read books, pored over tomes, watched videos about the power of positive thinking and healthy living. I may have been full of good intentions for a day or two, but then I had always reverted to my usual self before any action had been taken. I didn't need to be a rocket scientist to realise my first step in my battle was to equip myself with the means to fight. It was time for a radical change – starting with what I stuffed in my mouth.

Operation: Diet Overhaul was born on that patio, somewhere between the third and fourth beer:

Rule One: Vegetables. Real ones. Not the soggy garnish you push to the side of your plate. Actual, green, crunchy, nutrient-filled plants. Broccoli. Spinach. Carrots. Maybe even kale – though I drew the line at quinoa mainly because I had no idea what it was.

Rule Two: Fast food was out. Goodbye burger runs and fish and chips which could lubricate a tractor. Hello home-cooked meals – lean meats, fish which wasn't battered into oblivion, beans, lentils, nuts. Charlie swore these things were edible. I chose to trust her.

Rule Three: Sugar. My greatest frenemy. No more chocolate bars for breakfast. No more secret biscuit stashes. Charlie threatened to check my glovebox for contraband if she had to.

Rule Four: Beer. Not gone – let's not be barbaric – but limited. Moderation. A word I'd never practised, but there's a first time for everything.

Then came exercise – my least favourite word in the English language. I didn't mind walking so much, but we both knew I'd find every excuse under the sun, especially during a soggy WA winter not to do it. So the next morning, slightly dusty but weirdly clear-headed, Charlie frog-marched me into a fitness shop in Joondalup.

Treadmill or exercise bike – my poison of choice. I happened to verbally notice the price tags; she cut me off with a line that shut me up instantly:

"How much is your life worth?"

Point taken. I walked out the proud owner of an exercise bike I hated before I'd even pedalled it. Charlie bought it for me as an early Xmas present. Merry Christmas to me.

Most ideas cooked up while I'm drunk fall apart with daylight. But weirdly, this plan didn't. Over breakfast at our old café haunt – the one which kept us fed during the renovations when our kitchen was a war zone – we revisited every point. None of it sounded stupid. For the first time in a long while, something actually made sense.

When I finally pulled into her driveway back in Dongara, where her new life waited for her, I hugged her and made a promise: *I would never give up. No matter how hard this got, no matter how many times I fell apart, I'd get back up and fight.*

And Charlie knows one truth about me that cancer would soon learn the hard way: **I never break a promise.**

Going It Alone

I was barely out of Dongara and back on the highway heading south when negativity decided to climb right back into the passenger seat beside me. All the way north, with Charlie riding shotgun, I'd been a roaring, unstoppable force – ready to square up to cancer and knock its block off. After twelve years together, we'd tackled every mess life threw at us. Lose a job? No problem – tag team it. Financial headaches? Shoulder to shoulder. Fight me, fight her too. She was Batman; I was, well, Robin, trying to keep up. It was easy to be brave with Charlie's voice in my ear. Without it? Not so much.

The fear didn't creep in politely, either. It kicked the door down and brought its mate, Anger. I took it out on the car. Foot down, hands clenched on the wheel, I turned the highway into a racetrack. Every bend was a test of whether I secretly wanted to survive the next one. My brain replayed the same two lines like a scratched record: *I'm going to die! – Screw that, I'm going to win!* – back and forth, back and forth.

Just before rolling into Two Rocks, I did the only sensible thing a man in crisis can do: stopped off and bought another carton of beer. If last night's batch gave me courage, maybe tonight's could drown the fear again.

When I finally coasted under the carport, I could smell the brake pads hissing their disapproval. A four-hour drive done in just under three, with a bottle shop pit stop for good measure. Had I pinged any speed cameras? Almost certainly. Did I care? Not even slightly –

the postie could drop tickets for months. Cancer trumped fines.

On my knees at the fridge, I unloaded my new liquid shield onto the bottom shelf – prime position, obviously, because hot air rises and beer deserves the coldest spot. Science, don't argue. The sight of the other fridge inhabitants gave me pause: milk (innocent enough) and a collection of artery assassins which would give an ox a coronary if you baked them into a casserole.

I sat back on my heels, thinking about what lay ahead. Work wasn't the issue. I was self-employed, so I could scale up or down, take a day off to lie in a hospital bed, take two days off to cry under the Doona – whatever I needed. Money wouldn't kill me before the tumours did.

No, the real worry was my body – this poor, beer-fed, pie-powered machine. I was about to hand it over to the oncologists and tell them: *Do your worst, save what you can.* But the plan Charlie and I hatched over a carton of beer in the sunset stuck with me: *Don't just leave it all to the doctors.* If I wanted a chance, I had to get stuck in myself – front line, not the back seat.

Charlie's words from the night before rang in my skull:

"You have to be ready for that."

Meaning: if I kept feeding myself like a half-drunk teenager, I'd stand no chance once the chemo and hormone shots started waging war inside me.

Everything had to change. But not tonight. Not while my fridge still looked like an episode of *Kitchen Nightmares*. I'd gut it tomorrow – once I'd made a plan and stocked up on actual food which didn't come in a brightly-coloured box or cause heart palpitations just by looking at it.

That night, I knocked the cap off a fresh stubby, dragged a chair onto the patio, and watched the world shuffle by. My front table – my little fortress of calm – had always worked to settle my head. I'd watch cars crawl past, neighbours wave, the ocean roll in and out. But that night my thoughts bounced around my skull like a squash ball in a tin shed: positive, negative, positive, negative.

What's the point?

There'll be a cure any day now, right? I'll fight until then.

Will there ever really be a cure?

Can I handle months of torture just to buy more time?

Then Charlie's promise popped back up, full force: *I will never give up.* And I don't break promises. Especially not to her.

Beer number six (or maybe seven?) went the way of the rest. I swore tomorrow I'd gut the fridge, cycle a kilometre, eat a vegetable. Tonight I'd finish my beer and not think too hard about tomorrow.

One Day At A Time

Morning rolled around and the man staring back at me in the bathroom mirror barely looked familiar. Same face, same scars, but something behind the eyes – a stubborn glint which said:

"You said you'd fight. So fight."

On any normal day, I'd have hit the beach for my token walk – South Beach stretched for miles, enough to convince myself I was sporty while doing the bare minimum. But now there was an exercise bike waiting for me. Charlie had spent good money on it, so it was time to earn its keep.

I climbed on, full of purpose. Three minutes later, I was draped over the handlebars, gasping, convinced my heart was going to burst out my chest and decorate the spare room walls. How could I be this unfit? It was laughable. Except I wasn't laughing – I was crawling to the couch, trying not to pass out.

Once my pulse stopped sounding like a death metal drummer, I figured I'd do a press-up. One press-up. Easy. Right?

Ha! Down I went, palms flat, feet together. Up I pushed... a whopping forty centimetres. And then gravity claimed me – face first into the laminate floor. I lay there, checking if my nose was bleeding. It wasn't, so small win.

I gave up on being Arnie for the day, promising myself tomorrow I'd do four minutes on the bike and two press-ups. Baby steps, but steps all the same.

To salvage my ego, I threw on a jacket and went for a proper walk around the village. Walking was still my safe space – one thing I knew I could finish without needing an ambulance.

Back home, showered, the next big hurdle loomed: food. I was starving after my heroic attempts at fitness. I can't even remember what I cobbled together, but it probably should have come with a health warning. And then came the coffee dilemma.

One teaspoon of instant, a splash of full cream milk. Easy. Then I reached for the sugar. Habit. I froze. The new me wasn't allowed sugar. Not unless I wanted Charlie to materialise and slap it out of my hand.

So I pushed the sugar away and took a sip. Bitter. Horrible. Would my taste buds ever adjust, like they did when I first started smoking? Or was coffee about to become my next sacrifice? That decision would have to wait.

Shopping For A New Life

That afternoon, Google and YouTube turned into my survival guides. I scribbled down a shopping list which looked like it belonged to a health nut: broccoli, spinach, salmon, lentils and beans – things I'd never willingly eaten unless they'd been hidden in a burger.

At the supermarket, my routine – blitz in, grab beer and pies, blitz out – was dead. Now I wandered like a lost toddler, squinting at labels, pestering shelf stackers for help. Who Knew Shallots were onions? Not me.

Shopping took an hour and my trolley barely had anything in it. But I felt oddly proud.

Back home, my kitchen turned into a science lab. Steam this. Boil that. Don't set off the smoke alarm. Don't poison myself. Google and YouTube were saints. Slowly, it became edible – not Michelin-starred, but edible. Steamed broccoli, carrots, a piece of fish. Marginally better than heated cardboard - just.

A week in, I found honey at the back of the store – lifesaver! One teaspoon in my coffee and suddenly the bitterness was tolerable. Coffee survived another day. Win.

My new hobby of *not dying so soon* took over my days: researching vitamins, googling recipes, pedalling my bike while watching reruns of The Big Bang Theory. My press-ups climbed from one nose-plant to three and the count kept rising - slowly. The bike sessions crept up too – almost an hour, albeit on the same easy setting, but progress is progress.

Somewhere along the line, I realised something strange: during the day, the negative thoughts weren't as loud. They still popped up, but they didn't shout over everything anymore. Instead, my brain was too busy figuring out the difference between kale and spinach and how not to face-plant during push-ups. It was working. I was becoming more positive.

Charlie's voice came back: **"You need to be ready for that."** Maybe I wasn't bulletproof yet, but I was getting there.

Rebuilding More Than Myself

One problem I discovered on my journey into all things culinary: my tiny excuse for a kitchen was just that - tiny. When I was living on pies and takeaway, it did fine. Upending a cardboard box onto a plate required hardly any space. Now, with a chopping board, veggies and all this new *healthy nonsense*, the postage-stamp counter was driving me nuts.

So, out came the tape measure, sketch pad, and a mountain of swearing. One wall got moved, the laundry shrank to a broom closet, wires got rerouted, and slowly my shoebox of kitchen turned into a real cooking space. Double oven? Hell, yes! Do I need it? Not yet – but maybe one day.

Renovating gave me something to do with my hands and my head. When that project wrapped up, I found another. And another. Each hammer blow kept the dark thoughts at bay. I wasn't just rebuilding a kitchen; I was rebuilding me.

If You're Where I Was

If you're reading this because life's thrown you the same brutal curveball – here's my unsolicited advice: find yourself a project. Plant a garden. Learn to cook. Build a shed. Paint a mural. Whatever takes your fancy. Who cares if you don't finish it? It'll keep your head above the murky water when fear tries to drag you down. The more you are thinking about your project, the less time you have for negative thoughts to invade. The wrong thoughts will kill you faster than cancer will.

And above all else – keep your promises. Especially the ones you make to the people who stood beside you when you were too scared to stand alone.

On The Up

The rest of that carton of beer I bought after dropping Charlie back in Dongara was still chilling on the bottom shelf of my fridge. Once I kicked off my new diet and daily exercise routine, I swore off alcohol completely. Not forever – I'm not a monk – but after four decades of pickling my insides, I figured my poor liver deserved a bit of annual leave.

Days were getting easier. I'd start with a proper breakfast – not a leftover pizza or a soggy bacon sarnie, but actual food with vitamins and other goodies in it. Then I'd exercise and either go do a job for a customer or throw myself into a home project. Between researching healthy food and rebuilding my matchbox kitchen, my days were packed and, dare I say it, my general demeanour was becoming more upbeat as time wore on.

But come nightfall? Different story. As the sun clocked off for the day, my resolve started to subside. Darkness crept in, and my mental armour melted away like ice in summer. All the worries I'd wrestled into a corner during daylight came roaring back for Round Two the minute I sat still. I tried to reason it out: *Of course I'm going to get the wobbles – I've got bloody cancer.*

But then another theory sneaked in: maybe I wasn't just sad – maybe I was in withdrawal. Four decades of drinking like it was my hobby of choice, and suddenly – cold turkey. Perhaps my mind wasn't creating the problem, maybe it was my body pleading for the alcohol it had been accustomed to be soaked in.

Cue the nightly battle in my head:

One beer won't hurt. Don't be an idiot. One beer will make you feel normal. And what about your promise, genius?

I'd try to distract myself with a movie, but my mind didn't care what was on Netflix. It just wanted a beer – or failing that, a good cry. I decided I'd have to suck it up and hope my body eventually realised it wasn't getting drenched in lager every night and would stop sulking.

In the meantime, I doubled down on becoming Gym Bunny Lite. Within three weeks of *New Me*, I'd scored some cheap hand weights and a bench on Gumtree. Let's be clear: when I say *working out*, I'm not about to break any Olympic records. There's no "Eye of the Tiger" blasting while I sprint around Two Rocks high-fiving passing dogs.

I pedal my exercise bike at a pace your nan might manage while riding to bingo. I walk briskly, which is progress, and I'm up to ten press-ups a day – with no face-planting or emergency dental work required. With the new kit, I added chest flys, bicep curls, shoulder presses (a whopping seven kilos each, don't be jealous), and threw in the odd squat or burpee just to keep my heart guessing.

This new regime, plus my healthy eating, was fast turning Andy the Hot Mess into Andy the Not-Quite-a-Total-Mess. Sure, I knew I wouldn't be a ray of sunshine every second of every day – but if I spent more time being positive than negative, that had to be better than the alternative.

Mornings became a routine: wake up, eat something which didn't come in a greasy paper bag, shower, tackle the to-do list – repeat. The change in my demeanour was beginning to shine through. I felt hopeful about what I was trying to achieve. So good some days I caught myself thinking, *How the hell do I have Stage Four cancer?*

All I had to do was keep this up when the big guns started. Easy, right?

Chemo

Middle to late August rolled around, and it was time to pay my first proper visit to the Oncology Unit at Joondalup Hospital for Chemo Session Number One. I had six sessions planned, three weeks apart – a lovely six-pack of chemical warfare just for me.

I left home with plenty of time to spare. If the car broke down or a kangaroo protest blocked the highway, I didn't want to add a meltdown to my schedule. But halfway down the route to Joondalup, I started questioning my genius plan to drive myself.

What state would I be in after?

Would I be able to drive home? Surely they would have told me if I needed an adult to collect me... right?

Perhaps they did? Did I listen? Oh, shut up, Andy.

One thing I knew for sure: I wasn't paying those daylight robbery parking fees at the hospital. If I had to abandon the car overnight, I'd rather not need a second mortgage to get it back. So I parked at the shopping mall across the road – free – and enjoyed a five-minute stroll through the city sunshine toward my date with a chemical cocktail.

By the time the automatic doors whooshed open and I stepped into the pastel-painted, unnaturally bright reception of the Oncology Unit, I was absolutely petrified.

What were they going to pump into me? Would I puke my guts up? Would my hair all fall out at once? Why hadn't I Googled this shit?

The receptionist greeted me by name – Andy, not Andrew, because I'd filled in the forms properly. Instant gold star. I barely had time to sit before a nurse called Bronwen – all smiles and calm efficiency – emerged through the big double doors.

She introduced herself and whisked me off down bright corridors, stopping occasionally to weigh me (sure) and measure my height (less sure – is chemo going to shrink me to garden gnome size?). I'd already lost a few centimetres over the years; I couldn't afford to lose any more or people would start patting me on the head.

We reached the chemo ward and I braced myself for a torture chair. Instead, I found heaven. The thing they asked me to sit in looked extremely basic and very uncomfortable – more like a cheap office chair than a medical marvel – but the second my backside touched it, I knew I could sit there forever. No fidgeting, no numb bum, no backache. I mentally ordered one for my lounge room.

Bronwen hooked up bags of clear liquid and talked me through what would happen. She stuck a blue thingamajig into the back of my hand – painlessly, mind you – and attached tubes and drips like she was an electrician installing an electrical circuit.

One glance around the room reassured me: none of the other patients were foaming at the mouth or passed out. At least another 10 customers, some reading, some scrolling on their phones, none of them looking like a zombie extra from *The Walking Dead*. So I popped in my earbuds, fired up Netflix and pretended this was just another day at the spa – if spas offered poison in a drip bag.

Over the next hour, other nurses – Joanne, Jane, and a few more whose names I'd soon know well – came over to check on me. These women? Angels in scrubs. I can't imagine how they do it, surrounded every day by people facing the worst news life can hand out, yet still dishing out kindness and warmth with a grin. They have my utmost respect.

Time flew. One episode, maybe two, and Bronwen was back swapping out bags like a pit crew. I yanked out my earbuds, trying to look more alert than I felt.

"Just a quick flush and you're good to go!" she chirped.

Ten minutes later, I was free. No nausea. No fainting. Still with all my hair – for now. I walked back through the automatic doors into the sunshine, feeling more relief than fear for the first time in weeks.

Session one: done. Five more to go. Bring it on.

Side Effects

I retraced my steps back across the city under a clear blue sky, feeling ten feet tall and absolutely bulletproof. Whatever cocktail of chemicals they'd pumped into my veins at Joondalup that morning, the main bag might have been flushed through, but something was still fizzing away in my head – and it felt good. My mind was buzzing with so much positivity I was practically looking forward to Session Two.

A few days later? Well, reality came knocking – and it didn't bother to knock politely.

Slowly but surely, the side effects started to show up to the party, like those guests you invite but they never bring a bottle. To my mild surprise, the hair on my head stubbornly stayed put – but the rest of my body hair packed up and left. Even my short, once-proud goatee began to desert me in tiny grey drifts every time I rubbed my chin (something I do about a hundred times a day when I'm thinking). It wasn't painful – just weird. Same for my eyelids, which itched like mad but didn't actually hurt.

Next came the dull toothache – a loyal little bastard which popped up a day or two after each chemo session. It stuck around just long enough to make me reach for the painkillers, then vanished a couple of days later, only to return on repeat. A fun recurring guest star in my cancer sitcom.

By the second session, two more charming side effects clocked in for their shifts. First: my fingernails. They decided they'd had enough of being attached to my fingers. I kid you not – they started lifting. Technically, it was a build-up of pus between nail and skin slowly encouraging them to part ways after sixty-odd years of loyal service.

Now, most days that wouldn't be a huge issue. But I was still working part-time as a handyman, enough to pay my bills and keep my mind busy. And if you've ever worn denim jeans, you know their pockets aren't exactly generous – more like tight fabric clamps designed to infuriate. For decades, my pencil lived in my front pocket when not in use. No behind-the-ear nonsense for me – too awkward, too easy to lose.

So there I'd be, mind wandering, fingers diving into that tight pocket for my trusty marker. The second my fingertips hit the hem, my lifting nails would catch, press back the wrong way and – F###! Did it hurt? It hurt like hell itself.

Yes, I tried gloves. Ever tried fishing a stubby pencil out of a jeans pocket wearing gloves? Not possible unless you have fingers like knitting needles. I thought about wrapping my fingertips in band-aids, but I considered that they'd stick too well – changing them would mean ripping the nail off entirely, which felt a bit extreme. So I gritted my teeth and accepted that pocket pencils and loose nails were my new reality. For the record: I only lost one completely – my left pinky nail, which now lives in a tiny pill bottle in a drawer as a memento to my art and pain. Gross, but there it is. (And yes, a new one grew back.)

The other side effect was the big one – the one that

truly rattled me. It didn't hurt my hands or my teeth. It went for my mind.

The Darkest Side Effect

I was getting hit from both sides: Lucrin hormone injections every three months and chemo every three weeks. The hormone therapy started first, and after my first jab I noticed a few days of feeling low – proper miserable, acting a bit irrational. But I could rationalise it: *It's just the drug talking, Andy. You're fine.*

But when Lucrin and chemo teamed up? That low mood turned into something else entirely. Something darker than I'd ever known. For about five days, my brain crawled into a hole so black I could barely see a way out.

In that state, there was no reasoning. It never once occurred to me that the drugs were to blame. The drugs wouldn't *allow* that thought to cross my mind – they made sure I truly believed it was all me, my life, my hopeless future. They turned me from the mostly positive bloke fighting cancer into someone suicidal.

Yes, suicidal.

I started asking myself what was the point of dragging this out. The doctors had already told me my cancer was incurable. Why not control my exit? Beat it to the finish line before it stripped away every shred of dignity I had left? Those thoughts, as hideous as they sound now, made perfect sense in that black fog.

Somewhere in the depths of it, I called Charlie. If I'm honest, I think I was calling to say goodbye.

She knew me better than anyone on Earth. In twelve years, she'd never heard me talk the way I did that night

– broken, defeated, done. Worse for her, she was hours away by road, unable to rush over and shake sense back into me.

But she knew her best weapon: my word. She reminded me of the promise I'd made: *No matter how hard it gets, you don't give in.* The drugs had buried that promise under a ton of hopelessness – but she made me dig it up. She stayed on the phone, talking sense, fighting back against my nonsense until I promised her one thing: I'd call her the next morning. She hoped that tiny promise would still matter once the fog lifted.

I don't know how long that call lasted. I do know she probably didn't sleep a wink. And I'm sorry for that.

The morning as the sun rose, the darkness within me finally started to fade. I could remember every horrifying thought from the night before – but the drugs had let go of my brain. It was back in my control. I knew it was them, not me. Not something I could understand the night before. I felt foolish, embarrassed even, but also deeply grateful I hadn't done anything stupid.

I called Charlie. She answered on the first ring. Relief poured down the line from her end, and without scolding me once (though I deserved it), she made me promise – again – to ring her straight away if it ever happened again.

Of course, I agreed.

Did it happen again? Unfortunately, yes – same cycle, same chemical hell. Lucrin and chemo teamed up and dragged me back into that pitch-black cave where ending it all made perfect sense. Again, I rang Charlie. Again, she talked me down. If she hadn't... well, I don't even want to think about it.

Even now, it terrifies me how powerful those drugs were over my mind – how they convinced me every dark thought was my own, how impossible it was to reason that it was just chemistry. It makes you feel stupid once you're out of it. But when you're in it? You believe every ugly lie.

A WORD TO ANYONE FIGHTING THIS BEAST

This bit is really important:

If you have been diagnosed with cancer and you're going through chemo, hormone therapy, or any cocktail of treatments – tell someone you trust what might happen. Warn them. Make them promise to check in. Make yourself promise to reach out when your thoughts stop making sense.

You haven't lost your mind. It's the drugs messing with your wiring. You just need someone to remind you who you really are until the chemicals wear off and your brain is yours again.

It might save your life – the way Charlie saved mine.

Round Two

A week before my second chemo session, I did what would become routine: a blood test. The results got pinged to my GP and both my oncologists. Dr W, my calm radiotherapy wizard, was on holiday at the time, so his stand-in rang me. She told me her name, but she said it so fast I had no chance of catching it. That didn't matter – in my world, all doctors answer to "Doc" anyway.

She was a fellow Pom – which, if you haven't been to Australia, is how Aussies affectionately refer to us Brits. It was originally POHM and stands for *Prisoner of His (or Her) Majesty* – a nod to the days when Britain liked to export its least law-abiding citizens here for an extended camping trip. It always amuses me that they use the term of endearment so freely, considering so many Aussies today are proud descendants of those early troublemakers.

Anyway, this Doc rang just to check how I was faring with my new chemical companions. I pictured her skimming my file while we talked, probably looking for any sign I'd spontaneously combusted from all the drugs.

Then she paused.

"Wow!" she said suddenly. "You had this blood test done this week? That's dramatic!"

Now, if you're a patient with incurable cancer, the word *dramatic* from a doctor is enough to make you check your will. My heart practically left my chest.

Turns out, this was a *good* dramatic. My PSA – that

271

pesky little number which first screamed *You've got cancer, mate!* when it hit 13.4 – had just crashed down to 0.5. After one Lucrin jab and a single chemo session.

I was stunned.

"What does that mean?" I asked, probably sounding like I'd forgotten how English worked.

She reassured me it was all good news. Very good news. And when I hung up, my head was still spinning.

This Doc must have flicked through hundreds, perhaps thousands of files in her career. Does she say "Wow" every time? I doubted it. So maybe this result **was** unusual. And maybe – just maybe – my new diet, daily exercise, and accidental discovery of kale had helped too.

Ask an oncologist about this, and they'll tell you "No" faster than you can say quinoa. But I'll come back to that.

A few days later, I rolled up for chemo round two at Joondalup. This time, I parked right in the hospital lot – not because I'd won the lottery or suddenly become reckless with money, but because cancer patients get free parking. One small perk in an otherwise fairly grim loyalty programme.

After my first session, I'd scored the golden ticket: the earliest possible slot. 9:00 am in, 10:30 am out. Brilliant. I arrived early, flopped into a waiting room chair and prepared to reacquaint myself with the world's most comfortable chemo chair.

At 9:10, a nurse poked her head out, called my name – then Dr P's secretary, perched at her desk like a gatekeeper, jumped up.

"No, no! He hasn't seen Dr P yet!"

The nurse vanished back inside and I sat back down. And waited.

9:45 am rolled around. Dr P himself strolled in from outside – a solid forty-five minutes after my scheduled time. Maybe the delay was caused by him pausing to pick up a coffee and admire himself in a shiny shop window.

Ten minutes more for him to settle in and then, finally, he summoned me with that familiar sickly smile plastered on his face.

"Thank you for waiting," he said, all smooth politeness.

Like I had a bloody choice, you twat!

No, I didn't say it out loud. But I thought it loud enough to echo in my skull.

I sat in his plush leather chair while he flicked through my file.

"Wow!" he said.

Ah, so he'd just discovered my PSA result. Of course, in true Dr P style, he immediately chalked it up to the sheer brilliance of *his* chemotherapy. Lucrin? Diet? Exercise? My unbreakable spirit? Nah. All about Dr P. Genius at work.

He asked a few stock questions about side effects. I grunted out some answers, paid him seventy-five bucks for the privilege, then was waved back to reception to wait my turn for the drip bag. While I was waiting for my receipt, I counted at least ten more people lined up behind me – that's seven hundred and fifty. Not bad for less than a morning's "work", the first hour of which he was nowhere near his desk.

Andy, don't be cynical...

Session two was pretty much a rerun of session one. World's comfiest chair? Check. Nurses fussing like guardian angels? Check. Clear bags of poison? Check. Netflix to pass the time? Double check.

Then sunshine, fresh air, and feeling, bizarrely, like I could wrestle a crocodile if needed.

Each session after that ticked off like clockwork – more blood tests, more promising PSA numbers:

- Session Three: 0.2
- Session Four: 0.13
- Session Five: 0.11
- Session Six: 0.05

By session six, I was feeling so smug about that number that I finally asked Dr P the question which had been bothering me since the beginning.

"I was suspected of having cancer when my PSA was 13.4. At what number would you have said, *Nah, mate, you're fine*?"

He glanced at his chart, did the math for my age, and said, "About 4.2."

I stared at him. "So I'm at 0.05. Why am I still being treated for cancer?"

Oh, I was still riddled with it, apparently – it was just behaving nicely thanks to *his* chemo. Not a whisper about the Lucrin. Or my kale. Or the fact I'd basically turned into a monk on a treadmill with a green smoothie.

I paid him another seventy-five bucks on the way out. Dr W never charged me anything, by the way – his payment came straight from Medicare. Dr P? He got the Medicare payment too, but he clearly enjoyed filling up his little tip jar.

Session six wrapped up in mid-November 2020. I wouldn't see Dr P again until February 2021. Three months – an eternity when you've been living blood test to blood test.

So, naturally, at Christmas I pestered my poor GP for a blood test *just to check*. A couple of days later, she rang:

"All good. PSA's steady at 0.05."

Best Christmas present ever.

When February came, I had back-to-back appointments with Dr W and Dr P. Dr W was gentle, thorough, and explained that now chemo was done, the main job was to keep the little buggers asleep with the Lucrin. Dr P? He basically told me what I already knew, smiled his crocodile smile, and accepted his seventy-five bucks.

Dr W and I agreed there was no point paying Dr P to repeat the same words every few months. So I said goodbye to the chemo king (with no tears shed) and stuck with Dr W – especially since radiotherapy was still on the cards and that was firmly in his wheelhouse.

My February PSA was still 0.05. By my next check-up with Dr W in May, it dropped again: 0.02.

"Undetectable," Dr W said, beaming.

Turns out, the scale doesn't read anything under 0.02 – so technically, I could be sitting pretty at 0.01 or even lower. But until someone invents a fancier test, *undetectable* was good enough for me.

One thing I still ask myself: the chemo ended in November. I had only two more Lucrin jabs before May. So what made it drop from 0.05 to undetectable? Just the injections? Or was it also my rabbit food, the daily sweat sessions, and my refusal to crumble?

Ask an oncologist and you'll get the same polite shrug. They'll say no, of course. But you tell me: does it really sound like *just* the drugs did all that?

I have my answer. You can decide for yourself.

The Diet

(Or: **How I Stopped Eating Like a Student and Started Eating Like I Wanted to Live**)

By now, you've probably twigged that, at the time of my diagnosis, my well-being was about as robust as a paper straw in a pint of Guinness. Before all this medical mayhem kicked off, I'd never stopped to assess my mental, physical or emotional state. I assumed I was just... normal. You know, a solid 6.5 out of 10 on the Human Functionality Scale. Nothing dramatic. Nothing to write a memoir about.

Then came **The Verdict**. That quiet little moment when the oncologist hit me with words that I followed with "Oh." And Charlie, my rock, and part-time human reality check, backed it up with her own brand of gently-delivered truth bombs:

"The treatment's going to be *exhaustive*, Andy. You need to get your body ready."

Translation: "You're not Keith Richards. It's time to stop living like you've been marinated in lager and pork scratchings."

The penny dropped and my world shifted totally. I needed to get my act together. It was time for my body to start acting like it *wanted* to survive this rodeo. Which meant a radical overhaul of lifestyle, including the dreaded "E" word.

No, not "enlightenment."

Exercise.

Apparently, exercise not only helps you physically, but it stimulates the mind too. "Healthy body, healthy mind," they say, which is all well and good until your healthy body is screaming and your mind is begging for doughnuts.

Still, I gave it a go.

Now, let me take you back a few years to one of my FIFO gigs (that's "Fly In, Fly Out," not "Fast Inhale, Fast Out-of-breath," although that applied too). There I overheard an "ALC" (Active Life Coach) banging on about the power of exercise like he was auditioning for a Peloton ad.

But here's what stuck:

"Exercise only accounts for 20% of getting in shape. The other 80% is diet."

WHAT?! So, I could sweat myself into a puddle five days a week, but if I still stopped at the burger bar on the way home, it would all be pointless?

Charlie, bless her, bought me an exercise bike which looked like it could power a small village if pedalled hard enough. And thanks to a bloke on Gumtree who'd clearly given up on his New Year's resolution sometime around Australia Day, I snagged a gym bench and hand weights for fifty bucks. Bargain.

Exercise? Sorted.

But diet? Now that was a jungle.

I enlisted my trusty sidekicks: Google and YouTube. With a steaming cuppa and the determination of a man who's eaten his last sausage roll, I set off into the deep, unfiltered madness of the World Wide Web.

Previously, I had spent spare time clicking on YouTube with all the aimless enthusiasm of someone flicking through late-night telly. But this was different. This time, I had *intent*. I used the *search* button like a grown-up.

And what did I find? Chaos.

Apparently, every fruit-loop with a juicer, and an opinion has a YouTube channel. I was drowning in "Top 10 Superfoods That Will Literally Save Your Life" videos hosted by suspiciously shiny people who look like they've never eaten carbs or felt joy.

My poor mouse nearly exploded from all the frantic clicking.

How had so many idiots managed to cobble together a video which made no sense at all? I devised a vetting process.

Robotic voice? Gone.
Spelling mistake in the title? Goodbye.

Presenter claims bananas are a government conspiracy? NEXT.

All I wanted was facts. Is broccoli my friend or the devil in green florets? Does turmeric *actually* do anything or is it just curry glitter?

I was just about ready to give up and go back to eating toast for every meal when I stumbled across a video with a hint of promise – title spelt correctly, no robots involved – and a human being talking actual sense.

This guy wasn't shouting. He wasn't promising that

kale would make me immortal. He was just calmly explaining what foods fight disease, and why. Cruciferous vegetables, berries, whole foods – the gang was all there. And, shock horror, he had receipts. Science. Studies. Actual qualifications.

Ladies and Gentlemen, please allow me to introduce you to **Dr William Li** – my dietary Obi-Wan Kenobi.

This man is *everything*. Asian-American. Harvard-trained physician. Medical scientist. Walking talking academic mic drop. His credentials are so many, I'd need a separate appendix just to list them. I started watching all his videos. He was everywhere. Interviews, podcasts, online summits. And not once did anyone spell "nutrition" as "nutrashun." The more I saw, the more I knew I was going to be in safe hands if I adopted his advice into my diet.

I watched Dr Li for hours – some people binge Netflix, I binged disease prevention – and eventually discovered he'd written a book: **Eat to Beat Disease**.

Slam dunk. Amazon. One click. Done.

That book is now my food bible. It should be on the school curriculum, in hotel bedside drawers, and given out in waiting rooms instead of lollipops.

Armed with real knowledge (and a growing obsession), I started piecing together the big picture.

The deeper I dug into the research, the harder it was to pretend today's explosion of chronic illness was just some random cosmic prank. Spoiler alert: it's mostly our own doing–with a generous side-serving of corporate greed. Once upon a time, we ate to live. Sensible, right?

But somewhere along the way, that idea got flipped on its deep-fried head and we started living to eat... ideally things shrink-wrapped, deep-fried, or squirted from a novelty-shaped bottle.

We didn't see it coming. Too distracted by catchy jingles, buy-one-get-one-frees, and "NEW & IMPROVED!" labels slapped onto the same old processed nonsense. We marched – no, waddled cheerfully down a path to sickness, waving discount coupons in one hand and clutching a bucket-sized cola in the other, only to wonder years later how we ended up with six daily medications and a loyalty card for the pharmacy.

Back in the 1950s and '60s, people ate to live. These days, we live to eat. Somewhere along the line, the concept of nourishment was quietly replaced with slogans like "treat yourself!" and the marketing masterpiece that is "cheese-stuffed everything."

Let's rewind.

Once upon a time, local farmers actually grew real food in real soil that contained actual nutrients. They rotated crops. Every fourth year the fields got a break – agricultural long service leave – to recharge and restore the earth's vitality. Why? Because good soil equals good food, and good food meant your cells would practically high-five each other after dinner.

Now? Fields are worked to death like Victorian chimney sweeps. No holidays, no rest, just relentless extraction. The result? Soil with fewer nutrients than a stale popcorn kernel, and vegetables that look beautiful under supermarket lighting but are marginally more nourishing than a polystyrene sandwich.

So what happened?

Two words: the Sixties.

It was the decade of cultural upheaval and fabulous chaos. Everything became bold, bright, and rebellious. The Beatles and The Stones ruled the airwaves. Pirate radio broadcast from ships on the high seas. Mini-skirts, go-go boots, and long-haired men became the new normal. It was groovy, it was glamorous, and for better or worse, it changed everything – including how we ate.

Suddenly, eating became an event. Out went slow-cooked meals and in came TV dinners, tinned everything, and pre-packed convenience meals that looked like the future but felt more like a shortcut to something else entirely. Farmers were pressured to produce more, faster, cheaper. Mass production became the mantra.

Meanwhile, mums – who'd been running households like five-star generals – were called into the workforce to pay for all the shiny new "time-saving" must have appliances. Fridges meant food could last longer. But now that Mum was working 40 hours a week and still somehow expected to do everything else, there was no time to shop daily. Supermarkets sprang up, offering everything under one fluorescent-lit roof: meat, veg, milk, and 14 kinds of cereal your kids would beg for and hate by Thursday. The humble butcher and greengrocer – once pillars of the community – faded quietly into history.

Convenient? Absolutely.

Sustainable? Not exactly.

Nutritionally sound? Let's just say... not ideal.

And because we needed more food, from further away, and faster than ever, we got pesticides. Fertilisers. Chemical preservatives with names which sound like Bond villains. Processed food that looked amazing on a shelf but did bugger-all for your actual health. Add to that the rise of takeaway, ready meals, and sugar hidden in literally everything, and suddenly hospitals weren't just for births and broken limbs – they were filling up with people suffering from diseases we barely knew existed a generation ago.

Coincidence? Maybe.

Probable cause? You decide.

As for me? These days I look at a head of broccoli like it's a medicine cabinet in disguise. I know what "cruciferous" means – and no, it's not a spell from Harry Potter. Thanks to Dr Li, I've also learned that "anti-inflammatory" isn't just a posh way of saying "Panadol."

So if you take nothing else from this chapter, take this: food can be your friend, your medicine, or the thing which quietly tries to kill you over the course of thirty years. Choose wisely. And maybe – just maybe – eat the damn broccoli. Charlie was right. My body needed to start acting like it actually wanted to stick around.

Eat to Beat Disease by Dr William Li became my food bible. And I'll say this loud and clear: everyone should own a copy. It doesn't matter if you've been handed a diagnosis like mine – or if you're the picture of health. Prevention isn't just better than cure – it's cheaper, easier, and tastier. Seriously: buy it.

(The Serious Bit... with a Side of Steamed Broccoli)

Dr William Li's book isn't just a bedtime read – it's a deep dive into how everyday foods interact with your body's built-in defence systems to help prevent, manage, and in some cases, even reverse chronic diseases. And the best bit? It's all backed by real science, not some influencer's theory fuelled by celery juice and wishful thinking. Dr Li presents a compelling case for food as medicine – and not in the boring "eat your greens or else" way, but in a way which makes you think, *"Why didn't I know this before?"*

Speaking of which – here's a little wager I'd like to make: more than 95% of the people reading this book (wait, scratch that), more than 95% of the *entire human population* probably have no clue that the body has not one, not two, but **five** key defence systems. That's right – five unsung heroes working behind the scenes 24/7, and most of us treat them like a dodgy smoke alarm: we only notice them when they're malfunctioning.

So, in case you're not rushing off to buy the book just yet (you really should, but hey, free will and all that), here they are for your Googling pleasure:

- **Angiogenesis** - the body's way of growing blood vessels, which can help or hinder disease

- **Regeneration** - because your body can actually repair itself (who knew?)

- **Microbiome** - the good bugs in your gut that basically run the show

284

- **DNA Protection** - keeping your cellular blueprints from becoming chaos
- **Immunity** - your internal bouncer squad, working the door at Club You

And yes, if you do type those into Google, I guarantee Dr William Li's name will appear faster than a dodgy ad for "miracle detox tea."

Now, if you actually understand how these systems work and – crucially – give them a bit of a helping hand through what you eat, you're no longer just passively hoping for the best. You're actively stepping into the ring, gloves on, jabbing at disease before it even gets a chance to land a punch. And hopefully, avoiding the kind of diagnosis which came knocking at my door.

Enter: The 5x5x5 Framework

Also introduced in the book is Dr Li's *5x5x5 Framework* – a dead simple, practical guide which encourages you to eat health-supporting foods every day. That's five defence systems, five health domains, five food types. Most of these 200+ foods can be found right there in your local supermarket – not some obscure Himalayan super-root only available via smug influencers or monks named Kevin.

The problem? I had probably walked past them a hundred times.

"Oh look, it's got green leaves! Must be dangerous – quick, avoid eye contact!"

Not anymore.

Thanks to Dr Li, I finally started assembling an actual

diet plan, not just "whatever's in the fridge that isn't furry." My dinner plates now almost always include broccoli and carrots.

(I know, broccoli. I used to hate it too. Now it's basically my spirit vegetable.)

Let's take a moment for broccoli, shall we?

This unassuming green floret isn't just a side dish – it's a nutritional juggernaut. Vitamins A, K, B9, Potassium, Iron, Magnesium, Calcium, Fibre... plus a cast of hard-to-pronounce but incredibly beneficial antioxidants and phytochemicals like Sulforaphane, Lutein, Zeaxanthin, and Indole-3-Carbinol. All that goodness for a measly 31 calories per cup (raw).

And while I promised this book wouldn't turn into a science lecture, let me give Sulforaphane a quick shout-out. This compound has shown potential in fighting cancer by neutralising carcinogens and reducing inflammation. Basically, broccoli's wearing a cape and fighting crime at a molecular level.

Do I always eat clean? Not exactly.

I said "treat food as medicine" – not "live like a monk on kale and regret."

So yes, I still have the occasional KFC (herbs, spices... it *counts*), and once a week I throw some chips on the plate. But these are air-fried, not deep-fried, and they don't leave a film of grease on the plate that could lubricate a lawnmower.

My Kitchen Epiphany

Once my cancer journey got underway – and once I

stopped treating the kitchen like a foreign country – I invested in two appliances which changed everything:

- An air fryer with a steamer function
- A blender

The air fryer gets daily use, almost always in steamer mode. Why? Because steamed veg actually *taste* like food, not punishment. My previous cooking attempts produced results so bland, you could use them as insulation.

The blender was for smoothies – another revelation. Fruit, veggies, a splash of soy milk, and bam – I was blending my way into a new lifestyle. (Bonus: it also makes you feel oddly smug. Like someone who owns more than one yoga mat.)

So, if you've made it this far, congratulations. You've just had a crash course in nutritional common sense, backed by science, and filtered through the mouth of someone who used to consider barbecue sauce a nourishing food.

Eat well. Stay curious. Steam your veg. And trust me – your body will thank you in ways you never thought possible.

Radiotherapy

At the end of May 2021, Dr W set up a meeting at Genesis Care in Joondalup. He wanted to get serious about radiotherapy – something he'd hinted at nearly a year earlier when we'd first met at Charlie Gairdner's.

I arrived a bit early and sat pretending to watch the giant TV bolted to the wall. It droned out some forgettable daytime nonsense while I counted ceiling tiles and tried not to think too hard. True to form, right on the dot of 9 am, Dr W emerged from the consulting area. Third meeting with him – third time exactly on schedule. Why can't they clone him and send a version to train every other doctor in Australia?

Back in his office, he laid out the plan. If I agreed (which, at this point, I'd have agreed to having my head removed and reattached backwards if he'd recommended it such was my trust in the man), I'd start thirty-seven sessions of radiotherapy on June 2nd – Monday to Friday, seven weeks straight.

I nodded like an obedient schoolboy. Of course I agreed.

Before that could happen though, I'd need a minor bit of surgery. Dr V – the same delightfully bony-fingered surgeon I'd met earlier in my prostate-poking saga – would pop in some gold "seeds" inside my prostate. These would help the radiotherapists pinpoint the little bugger with millimetre accuracy.

Locate my prostate? I nearly laughed. Dr V had found it just fine before, thank you very much – no GPS required, just her knuckles of steel. But apparently, in the world of precision radiation, a few gold nuggets stuffed up your backside make everything easier to aim at.

Bonus: general anaesthetic! I do love a nap I don't remember taking. Plus, post-op, I'd be technically worth more at the scrapyard.

Along with my new internal bling, they'd tattoo a few dots on my hips – so the team could line me up perfectly on the machine each session. Easy enough to follow, even for a thicko like me.

Once the science bit was explained, Dr W asked how I was holding up in general. I told him the truth: fewer dark days, healthy food, exercise, and honestly, it still felt impossible that there was anything wrong with me at all. Was he *sure* I had cancer? He was.

Then he perked up about something new: a free gym program at Genesis Care. The machines were brand new, a personal trainer would tailor everything to me, and research suggested staying active could reduce the crushing fatigue radiotherapy tends to bring. He seemed genuinely excited about it – so of course, I signed up on the spot. If Dr W had told me tap dancing lessons would help, I'd have dusted off my jazz hands.

To top it off, I was assigned a personal radiotherapy nurse – Julie S. She was my living, breathing Google for anything radio-related. Any question, any worry, she'd answer it (and if she didn't know at the time of me asking, she'd find out and ring back pronto). Twice I called her with random panics, and both times she not only sorted me out but had me howling with laughter. If

Julie ever fancies a career change, stand-up comedy would be her calling.

A couple of days later, I returned to Genesis Care for my first chat with Pam, the personal trainer. Same carpark as before, but this time instead of hitting "3" for Dr W's office, I'd been told to press "B1" – gym level.

I stood at the lift wondering what sort of architectural clown names a floor *B1* when I was already in the basement. Was this a prank? Nope – turns out I wasn't just in the basement – I was about to descend *under* the basement. Deep enough that if they'd dug a bit more they'd have hit the Earth's core or at least an old lava flow.

Sure enough, the lift lurched lower, doors opened, and there I was: face to face with a hand sanitiser dispenser and a stern sign about wearing a mask (Covid rules – still alive and well). I scrubbed my hands, masked up, and followed the corridor until I found the reception.

I plonked myself in another supremely comfy chair, admired the stale magazine selection, and sipped at the free coffee I'd been offered by the smiling staff. It was then I realised what was bugging me: *no windows*. Of course there weren't – we were buried so deep underground that sunlight had long given up trying to find us. It made sense, though – if they were going to blast people with radiation daily, better to keep it down here rather than next to a childcare centre.

I spotted two ominous passageways leading off into the gloom. Now I knew: that's where the actual zapping happened. I stared at them like they might roar to life and swallow me whole.

"Andy?" snapped me back to Earth.

Pam, the personal trainer, impossibly fit and cheerful, greeted me and whisked me through yet another corridor into the gleaming gym.

We spent a half hour going through my self researched exercise history and measuring bits I'd rather not think about. She got me to test some equipment so she could design my personalised sweat torture. By the time I left, we had a plan: when radiotherapy started, I'd be training here like a champ – unless I grew an extra limb from the radiation first.

The gold seeds were planted by Dr V without drama (I suspect she enjoyed rummaging around in there). My plan to break in the gym before treatment fizzled out – too much driving back and forth from Two Rocks to Joondalup. So I stuck to my home routine and promised myself I'd use Pam's gym once the daily zapping started.

And then – day one of thirty-seven.

Half an hour before leaving home, I chugged exactly 375 millilitres of water – the magic number for my bladder size. Not too empty, not too full.

I parked up, descended once more into the radioactive underworld, masked up, sanitised, and was greeted by the ever-sparkling Sarah and Deb at reception. Coffee? Declined. My bladder was locked and loaded – I wasn't about to risk overflow before the lasers hit me.

Soon enough, a young therapist (new face) appeared from the dark corridor and beckoned me in. She made cheerful small talk as we walked: Did I drink the water? How was I feeling? She clearly spotted the deer-in-headlights vibe.

Inside the treatment room – bigger than expected, minimal furniture, but dominated by a machine the size of a small truck. It looked a lot like a CAT scanner, except this one didn't slide *me* in and out. Instead, the big spinning bit whirred around *me* while I lay perfectly still, hip tattoos exposed to the world.

Monica and Dan fussed over my position until my gold seeds and hip tattoos lined up just so. They dimmed the lights – spa vibes – and piped in some 80s music.

"Relax and enjoy," Dan said with a grin as they left the room and the machine hummed to life.

Ten minutes later, lights back up, Monica and Dan reappeared and congratulated me. Session one done. Honestly? After chemo, radiotherapy felt like a day at the beach: lie down, listen to music, go home. How on Earth does anyone get fatigue from that?

I found the loo fast, liberated my precisely measured 375ml, then – feeling oddly smug – headed for the gym.

The Bell

The gym at Genesis Care wasn't just rows of shiny machines and the occasional overenthusiastic grunt. Pam's workout plan for me was almost identical to what I'd cobbled together at home, so technically I could have skipped their gym entirely, and done my sweat sessions back in my own tiny house.

But if I'd done that, I'd have missed out on one of the greatest surprises of my cancer adventure: the people.

Tracey, Robert, Don, Carol, Glenn – and others whose names drift back to me now like warm echoes. Each one an absolute gem of a human. There's a magic which happens when you're in a room full of people who are fighting the same battle you are – no explanations needed, no pity parties, just instant camaraderie and a shared sense of humour which could make even the darkest days feel lighter.

Funny thing – we never really talked about our cancer. Not the grim details anyway. But we laughed – a *lot*. The jokes which bounced around that gym floor were worth more than all the fancy machines. Because of them, and because of Pam, I kept going back to that basement bunker of sweat and giggles long after my radiotherapy officially ended.

And it wasn't just my gym crew. The staff on B1, the whole merry gang, became more than support workers. Over those weeks, they quietly morphed from friendly professionals into real friends – and by the time I was nearing the end, they felt like family. The good kind, not the ones you dodge at Christmas.

About halfway through my sessions, Dr W called me upstairs for a quick check-in on Level 3. He wanted to see for himself how I was faring. It was classic Dr W: calm, unhurried, genuinely interested.

He asked how I was feeling. I told him the truth: I'd done twenty out of thirty-seven sessions, and I didn't feel tired at all. In fact, I was still working every day – some days I'd finish up in Pam's gym, get changed in the downstairs bathroom, then head straight to a job site south of Joondalup. I was basically unstoppable. And Dr W seemed quietly chuffed about that.

And it all stayed that way until about session twenty-nine.

It wasn't so much exhaustion at first – more an increasing urgency to locate the nearest toilet. Fast. The time between *Hmm, I need a pee* and *Oh dear, that's happening right now* got shorter and shorter. My little house, for once, turned out to be a blessing: no matter where you stand, you're never more than five paces from the bathroom.

Strangely, the journey to Joondalup with my bladder brimming with its ritual 375 mils never caused me grief. But after session twenty-nine, instead of heading for the gym after the zap, I'd make a beeline for the bathroom, then straight home. Sleep started claiming bigger chunks of my afternoons, and for the first time, the famed radiotherapy fatigue caught up with me. The staff were amazed I'd gone as long as I had without feeling it.

Those final sessions squeezed every drop of fight out

of me. On my last day, after that thirty-seventh round of invisible laser punishment, I was done. Completely, utterly, no-more-left-in-the-tank done. If they'd told me, *"Oops, Andy, we miscounted, just one more to go,"* I'd have shaken their hands, politely refused, and crawled to my car.

Halfway down the corridor on B1, on the way back to the lift, there's a big bell bolted to the wall. Its purpose is simple and beautiful: when you finish your final treatment, you grab the rope and you ring that bell loud enough to shake the dust from the ceiling.

And when it rings, everyone stops. Whether they're waiting for their session, sipping coffee at reception, or mid-burpee in the gym – they clap. They clap like maniacs. Because they know exactly what it took for you to reach that rope.

Even now, recalling it makes my eyes sting. Writing this, I can feel my throat tighten the same way it did that day.

I walked up to that bell, drained but weirdly buzzing inside. I grabbed the rope, gave it a mighty pull – and it rang. Loud. But not as loud as the applause which erupted behind me. Patients, staff, my gym family – all clapping, all smiling with that fierce, kind look people get when they've watched you fight and win a battle they know too well.

I'd promised myself I wouldn't turn around – just ring it, keep walking, get in the lift, get on with life. But of course I turned. I looked. I saw them all standing there, clapping, laughing, crying with me.

And my tears – the ones I'm blinking away even as I write this – flowed just as freely then.

That bell didn't mean *cured*. It didn't mean *done forever*. But it meant I'd faced it, all of it, and I was still here to ring the bloody thing.

And for that, there will never be enough thank-yous to my gym crew, my B1 family, or Dr W and his magnificent army of angels.

The Letter

A couple of days before my last radiotherapy session, I had been early for one of my appointments and had sat patiently in the waiting area. With nothing to do but look around, I spied a cork wallboard I hadn't noticed before. Pinned to it were a plethora of 'Thank You' cards. They had all been sent by patients who, like me, were all grateful for the amazing care they had received from the staff of Genesis Care.

I had been so wrapped up in making sure I got to the bathroom before pissing my pants in the last week, thanking everyone for looking after me so well had completely slipped my mind. I knew I too had to find a way to say Thank You.

If I bought a card, it would, no doubt, be pinned to the same notice board by either Sarah or Deb, the two receptionists. Would all the staff get to see what I had written inside? I had no idea.

Perhaps I could get around that question by giving them all separate Thank You cards. But not all the same staff worked on the same days. They would be hard to distribute with only a couple of days to go.

I settled on the idea of an email, and I would ask for it to be printed out and left where all the staff were guaranteed to see it.

This is a copy of that email.

Hi, to each and every one of you marvellous people at Genesis Care.

As my treatment nears completion, I wanted to write and pass on a few thoughts which have come to mind during my time in your care.

I don't mind admitting, at the outset, I was fearful. No, let me rephrase that, I was downright terrified. On a scale of 1 to 10, I was bubbling around 15. However, those feelings slid down the scale somewhat after my initial chats with Julie S***** who, in the short term, managed to bring the fear factor down to a more manageable 5 or 6. But as the big day loomed, the thought of spending time in a 'one-seater microwave' was sending my blood pressure north again, so to speak. Suddenly everything Julie had told me to allay my fears, flew out of the window and I was surrounded in a thick, seemingly impenetrable cloak of fear again.

I remember Day 1 quite clearly. Heading down to the lowest level in the lift for treatment seemed strangely appropriate. The road to Hell goes down, right?

Somehow I made it to the reception desk. God knows how, because with every step I was sure I was going to turn around and 'do a runner'. But that was the point where everything began to change, starting with the welcoming smiles of Deb and Sarah which would put the most agitated person at their ease. You both had the most calming influence on me. Some might say you are trained to do this. I don't believe that. You either have it or you don't. And you both have it in spade loads.

Then I started to meet the Treatment and Exercise Clinic staff. What an amazing bunch of people! In truth, the word

AMAZING does not begin to cover it. You are absolutely awesome! And every one of you possess a quality I find difficult to put into words. I'm going to call it 'Je ne sais quoi' (French for a quality that cannot be described or named easily).

I have been to many places where staff treat you with kindness, but more often than not, they do it because it is in the manual, it's their job. I often liken those experiences to those American movies where the young couple turn up in a town which isn't on the map and everyone is so nice, you just know something isn't right. Definitely NOT SO at Genesis Care. Everything IS right and EVERYONE genuinely cares. Over the last 7 weeks, I have been treated like royalty whilst being made to feel like a long-term friend. To do that you have to possess 'Je ne sais quoi'.

Remember my first day? Full of fear? Well, that only lasted for the first 10 minutes.

Everybody involved at Genesis Care saw to that. That day, after my first treatment, I walked out of B1 smiling and wondering what I made all the fuss about. The next few weeks no longer seemed daunting and that was because Genesis Care employs totally awesome, amazing individuals who possess 'Je ne sais quoi'.

As earlier mentioned, my treatment is coming to a close, and whilst I suppose ending the treatment is a good thing, it is tinged with some sadness as I honestly do enjoy being around you good people of Genesis Care. You are all the kind of people I would like to associate with. I will continue to use the Exercise Clinic for some time, but I will miss those 2-minute chats we had as you walked me into and out of treatment. I will miss your smiles and I will miss the JE NE

SAIS QUOI that every one of you possesses. You are all truly amazing.

As I sign off, I want to thank you from the deepest reaches of my heart for all the kindness, courtesy and outstanding professionalism you have all afforded me, I know I will never ever be able to repay you for everything you have done for me. Thank you. Thank you. Thank you.

With honest affection for you all,

Andy Partington

I thought long and hard about adding this email to the book. After all, it was a personal message to the fantastic staff of Genesis Care, Joondalup. The reason I did copy and paste it here is as follows.

About a week after I finished my last session of radiotherapy, I attempted to go back to the gym. I wasn't ready, but I was missing my B1 friends. As I reached reception, I was greeted by Sarah and Debs. They both thanked me for what I had written in what they said was a 'beautiful' email.

I smiled and told them it was just me saying 'thanks'. Then they went on to tell me what happened to my email.

Debs, after making sure all the staff had seen it, had forwarded it to Head Office. Whoever read it there, passed it along the chain, all the way to the top.

From there it came back down and found its way into the press office who also organised and edited the monthly newsletter distributed throughout Genesis Care, Australia.

So if my clumsy thank you could brighten a staff room *and* a corporate newsletter, it can live here too – for anyone who needs reminding that kindness never goes unnoticed.

Post Treatment

Two weeks after radiotherapy ended, I decided I was ready to go full Rocky Balboa and hit the gym properly. I'd actually tried the week before – bless my deluded optimism – but after fifteen minutes (if that) on a treadmill, my body had other ideas. Those ideas included collapsing like a pensioner on a pogo stick.

Drenched in sweat and gasping like a fish on a footpath, I stuffed my workout sheet back in the drawer, grabbed my phone and keys, and shuffled toward the exit of B1, looking for all the world like a fat kid denied entry to a burger joint. I passed a few desks – admin staff, nurses, assorted lovely humans – and gave them a weak wave or half-smile as I lurched by.

I was almost home free, heading toward the lift, when a nurse at the final desk spotted me. Her warm smile dropped quicker than my blood pressure, and in one smooth move, she leapt up, intercepted me like a linebacker, and frogmarched me into a side treatment room.

"Sit!" she barked, pointing at a chair with the kind of authority usually reserved for military police or disappointed grandmothers.

Moments later, I had probes stuck to me, a cuff cutting off circulation to my arm, and a full interrogation underway. Fortunately, after a couple of minutes, the gadgets blinked back the right answers. Nurse Interrogator released me with strict instructions: drink water, rest, and – under no circumstances – do anything remotely resembling exertion for 24 hours. Message received, Commander.

That's GenesisCare for you – they really do care. If they see something even slightly off, they don't ignore it.

A week later, I gave the gym another go. This time, I made it through my entire workout. I was knackered, sure, but I did it. And like the proud idiot I am, I took this as the universe giving me the green light to go back to work. I thought my body had fully recovered from the radiotherapy.

I remember someone, somewhere, during the flood of advice I received, telling me that recovery from cancer treatment can take months – sometimes years. Pfft, what a load of tosh! Or so Mister Clever Clogs Andy Partington thought. I was sure I was fit as a fiddle after only two weeks. If only hindsight was foresight. And if only I wasn't as stupid as I can often be.

The beauty of being self-employed is flexibility. I could squeeze in a gym session before heading off to fix someone's tap, door, or whatever domestic crisis they were facing. At first, it was a bit of a slog – shorter days, slower pace – but within the week, I was back to my old self.

Actually, scratch that – my *new* self. Let's not glorify the old me. Old Me? Thought a nutritious dinner came in a paper bag stamped "Macca's" and beer counted as hydration. New Me? He was into vegetables. Real ones. Not frozen or deep-fried.

I was exercising. I was eating like an adult. I was working, fixing up the house, and for the first time in decades, I was feeling genuinely good about myself. Stage Four cancer and all, I'd somehow landed in a place where I was... okay. Most of the time, anyway.

With treatments behind me, I believed I was recovering fast – physically and mentally. So *I* thought.

Once my initial fury at the universe and everyone in it had simmered down, and the "Why me?" sob story had run its course, I started thinking about the friends I'd lost over the years to accidents, suicides, and chronic illnesses. Too many and far too young. Chris in a car crash. Leroy and John M to suicide. Paul D in a fire. Paul S to cancer. John E's heart gave out. John T was fatally stabbed. The list goes on: Sharon I, John A, Lyn P... Too many names. Too many stories cut short.

Of everyone I've just mentioned, only two made it past sixty. Meanwhile, here I am at sixty-five, moaning about a terminal illness like some kind of whinging miracle. Statistically, I'm ahead. Could cancer eventually take me out? Sure, and at some point it probably will. But so could a runaway ute the next time I cross the road. Perspective, my friends. It's powerful stuff which goes along way in the pursuit of a positive attitude.

Sure, I still have my wobbly moments – but they are becoming fewer and further between. And when they do show up, usually for a few days after a Lucrin jab, they rarely stay long. Positivity was beginning to reign once more.

In the early days of the "Why me?" spiral, something Barbara T said planted a seed. It made me wonder if the universe wasn't punishing me, but warning me – offering a nudge rather than a curse.

Barbara and her husband Ian are my longest-standing customers of the Handyman business, and have become dear friends. They have three sons – one of whom works in cancer research – and somewhere along the way, I seemed to have become their honorary fourth. No extra chores, thank God.

When I arrive at their place, the first 30 minutes are always the same: Ian makes tea, and we sit around putting the world to rights. We call it "pre-job planning," but really, it's just catching up. The actual work starts... eventually.

One morning, I was telling them how I'd flipped my lifestyle: daily walks, leafy greens, less alcohol, fewer near-death takeaways. Barbara just nodded and said, "Do you think cancer came as a warning sign, not a death sentence? It's certainly made you change how you live."

Boom. Brain freeze. I just sat there blinking.

She wasn't wrong. She even added – gently – that I looked a hell of a lot better than when I used to rock up smelling like cigarettes and last night's regrets.

Barbara and I have had plenty of cosmic chinwags over the years – about the universe, fate, all that spiritual jazz. We're no Hawking and Sagan, but her question stuck.

Was cancer the universe's way of saying, "Oy, change course or die"? Had I stayed on the Macca's-and-full-strength highway, would I already be a memory with a beer named after me?

Looking back, the answer's probably yes.

Earlier, I said I was okay with having cancer. I meant it. Mostly. But as my mate Louise likes to put it, I still had my "wonky" days.

I'd been through chemo and radio and somehow come out the other side relatively intact. I thought I'd bounced back fast – working again within a fortnight, like some kind of medical overachiever. But it took me a couple of years to realise just how *not* recovered I actually was.

The reality is: chemo and radio happened in neat, defined chunks. First one, then a break, then the other. I thought the breaks were just hospital admin juggling calendars. Nope. They were mercy recesses. A chance for my body to catch its breath between batterings.

And all the while, lurking in the background like a hormonal boogeyman, was Lucrin. Started in July 2020, jabbed every three months since – and unlike chemo and radio, it wasn't going anywhere. Long-term tenant. No plans to vacate.

Once again, I underestimated it.

It was only with hindsight – and a few raised eyebrows from people aware of my situation – that I began to see a pattern in my post-jab weirdness. Turns out, a few days after a Lucrin injection, I had a tendency to go a bit... off-piste. Sometimes it was a dip into depression. Other times, I'd talk in riddles and wonder why nobody understood my very logical decision to alphabetise the dog food in Woolies.

In late 2021, during one of those "wonky" spells–

Louise's favourite term – I called Charlie. Because of course I did.

These dips weren't as black as the terrifying holes from late 2020, when chemo and Lucrin were tag-teaming like the villainous duo from an emotional WWE match. But I still struggled. I couldn't picture a future. Cancer felt like a shadow cast over every plan.

And yet – despite all that – I still believed, and still do, that a positive attitude is the only way to live. If you have cancer, you're better equipped to fight it. If you don't, it's still a damn good way to live.

Charlie didn't have a psychology degree. She didn't need one. She made sense. In the middle of my spirals, she anchored me. One conversation and I'd go from existential void to "What's for dinner?" She had that gift – shining a torch into the cave and pointing out the ladder I couldn't see. And bless her, she never demanded promises. She just helped me find the light – then probably needed a stiff drink and a nap.

Not every jab sent me to the emotional basement. Sometimes it just made me weird. Like, "let's build a backyard submarine" weird.

On those days, I'd have ideas which sounded brilliant in my head. Unfortunately, they translated to things like:

"I just need a plunger, three coat hangers, and a dolphin emoji – I think I can fix the housing crisis."

To the rest of the world: gibberish. To me: borderline genius.

When I explained this to a female friend, she just

smiled and said, "Sounds like me every month."

And that, ladies and gents, was the day I retired from making jokes about women's monthly cycles. Respect.

A few months after radiotherapy, I was still running my handyman gig when the siren call of FIFO life started echoing again. I was working alone, living alone – and while I was feeling better each day, I missed having someone to talk to. Not about cancer – just *talk*. Normal, everyday chatter. Even a weather conversation would've done wonders.

Just as I was weighing it all up, fate stepped in – disguised as a phone call.

It was Andrew B, a mate from the Roy Hill Mining Village days. He and his wife Kaila were a couple Charlie and I instantly clicked with. They've known about my situation from the start and have always been incredibly supportive. Best of all, they treat me like I don't *have* a medical condition.

"You want a maintenance role up in Pannawonica?" Straight to the point, as ever.

I did. But would my cancer history kill the opportunity before it left the ground?

He didn't think so. Said if the site doc passed me fit, the job was mine.

And two weeks later, I was back in high-vis, elbow-deep in Pilbara dust, cracking jokes in a crib room with a bunch of sparkies, plumbers, and fridgies – all armed with the kind of dry humour which should come with a warning label.

The work was hard. Twelve-hour shifts in up to punishing 50 C Pilbara heat, quite often without a whisper of shade. And yes, you read that correctly: *50 degrees Celsius*. That's not a typo. That's a slow roast.

But the banter kept things light, and during the day, my mood was solid. It was the nights which got to me.

No matter how hot the day had been or how exhausted I was, I rarely managed more than five or six hours of sleep. Which left me with around five hours of unstructured, dangerous time... the kind where your brain wanders into places it shouldn't.

Back home, I had creature comforts – my music, my half-finished DIY projects, a guitar, a keyboard, my design software. A thousand ways to occupy myself.

On site? I had a windowless room with all the charm of a dentist's waiting room – minus the out-of-date magazines. It had a bed, a fridge, a TV, an en-suite, and Wi-Fi which worked about as well as an inflatable dartboard. There was a bar on site, sure, but I didn't want to slide back into old habits – even if the beer was practically free.

One evening, while contemplating another thrilling night of showering, Netflix buffering, and pretending to enjoy Candy Crush, I noticed a laminated village map stuck to the back of my door. I'd opened that door at least three times a day, but somehow never saw it. Suddenly, inspiration struck.

At 3:00 a.m. the next morning, I was up. By 3:05 a.m., I was walking into the nearest site gym. To my surprise (and relief), it had everything I was used to at Pam's gym back in B1. So, my routine could stay the same. Familiar pain is still pain, but it's better than reinventing the torture wheel.

Later that day, I drove my glorified golf buggy – my official work vehicle – around the outer ring road and estimated the loop at around two kilometres. Three laps and I'd kill another hour. Combine that with the gym, and I could drown out any creeping negativity with endorphins and sore calves.

So that was it. End shift. Into my cell. Track pants on. Out for my walk. Dinner. Netflix or Candy Crush. Rinse and repeat.

And it worked. I had just enough on my plate to keep the gloom at bay. No time for existential dread when your legs ache and your back's threatening to form a union.

Still, in those early days, I had doubts. Had I made the right choice diving back into FIFO life? Especially now, older, and – well – technically radioactive.

But then something strange and wonderful happened.

Actually, **three** things happened.

Event 1

When I first took the role as General Hand / Handyman, the roster was your standard FIFO fare: two weeks on, one week off. Not ideal, but workable. Then came a twist worthy of a Hollywood rom-com – after some back-and-forth between the client company and the one I was working for, they flipped the roster to *one week on, one week off*. No reduction in pay. Same coin, half the grind.

That's not a pay rise, that's a **23% pay rise** and a massive upgrade in quality of life. It meant every second Thursday I was either heading home to sanity, or getting ready to check in for just seven days in my air-conditioned cell block. Happy bloody days.

But wait... there's more.

Event 2

On one of my returns to site, I wandered into my room expecting the usual "wiped over with a damp rag" level of clean. Instead, I walked into what felt like a hotel suite which had just passed a five-star inspection.

The air smelt... fresh. The floors gleamed. The bed looked like it had been styled by a wedding planner. It wasn't renovated – just immaculately cleaned. And not the usual "mining village clean", but proper, obsessive-compulsive, mum's-coming-over kind of clean.

On the bed, the usual little "cleaned by" card. This time: **Jayde**.

Who was Jayde? I had no idea, but whoever she was, she clearly needed to be cloned and deployed across every mining site in Australia. I made a mental note to thank her – just as soon as I figured out which housekeeper she actually was.

During my previous swing, I'd run into a glitch on the job: a work order came through on my tablet about mould creeping along the edge of a shower tray.

Apparently, it had sunk so deep into the silicone that no amount of industrial-strength spray or prayers could shift it.

No worries – I could sort the problem out. One small snag: the work order was missing a room number. No location. Just a mouldy mystery.

We had 800 rooms on site. I wasn't going to opt for Option 1. Ring head office and spend 40 minutes listening to hold music which sounded like it was composed by a drunk robot. Option 2 was also a route I didn't want to take - Delete the problem from the tablet and swear it was never there. Not my style. So I settled for Option 3. Ask the housekeepers.

Housekeepers, without any shred of doubt, are the unsung heroes of every mining village. They clean, they lift, they scrub. I certainly believe they are the hardest workers on any mine site.

When they're not being cleaning ninjas, they huddle in shaded pergolas and have a well-earned break. And they deserve every second.

So, I found a cluster of them gathered under one such pergola and rolled up in my buggy like the world's slowest cowboy.

I asked the question: "Any of you know about mould being reported in a shower tray?"

A few of them turned around.

Wow!

One of them had *that* smile. A smile I hadn't seen for over thirty-five years. It was one which instantly reminded me of someone I hadn't seen in decades – **Nikki T.** A soft, knowing grin which had once been a fixture of my life in the '80s. I'd never forgotten it.

"It was me," said the Nikki-smile-alike.

She remembered the room number, I thanked her, and drove off... still a bit stunned. For the rest of the day, I found my mind wandering back to Nikki. What was she up to? Was she still in Bridgend? Was she happy? The last I heard she was married with a couple of kids. We'd drifted apart too easily. Back then, it only took one missed weekend and a new job to fall out of a whole friendship group.

Years ago, I'd even tried to find her on Facebook. But I only ever knew her maiden name, and she used to spell her given name **Nicky**, not Nikki. She had exited the scene so quietly I never knew who she'd married. Every digital trail ended in a dead end.

Fast forward a swing, and I'd just returned to site, ready to work through my usual backlog of maintenance issues. Driving around the ring road, I spotted the Nikki smile again – same housekeeper, heading into a room.

I pulled up.

"You're Jayde, right?" I asked.

She smiled. That smile again. Bingo! She was the one who had cleaned A9, my room, with the kind of precision which makes surgeons weep with envy.

I thanked her profusely. Laid on the praise thick. She looked genuinely surprised–probably because housekeepers rarely get thanked, despite doing the work which keeps the whole show running.

From that point on, it was like she was everywhere I was. I bumped into her constantly. At one point I even joked, "You stalking me?"

She laughed. Then, during another encounter, she got a bit cheeky.

"I've seen you walking around the village at night," she said. "Trying to lose weight? Or just keeping fit?"

I explained my evening routine – three laps, good for the head. She nodded thoughtfully.

"I'm trying to stay fit too. Mind if I join you?"

What could I say? I was a polite bloke. I said yes.

Then walked away wondering what the hell I'd just agreed to.

Jayde looked about nineteen. Maybe twenty. I half expected her to show up for the walk still clutching a Barbie and wearing glitter shoes. The last thing I wanted was to spend my post-shift cooldown hour chatting with someone who might not even remember the Spice Girls as anything more than a Spotify recommendation.

I could've said I preferred walking with music. I could've said I needed the solitude. But I didn't. So I braced myself for one long, awkward hour.

At 6 p.m., in track pants and low expectations, I showed up. And then so did she. And within two minutes –*I was wrong*. So, so wrong.

Jayde was clever, sharp, and genuinely funny. She had the kind of dry wit which hit you sideways and left you gasping for air from laughing. We walked the village three times. Maybe four? I lost count somewhere between belly laughs.

After the walk, we headed into the dry mess for dinner, chatting like old friends. By the end of the night, when we split at the path between our rooms, she turned to me:

"Same time tomorrow?"

And just like that, our nightly walks became a thing.

It has been said that "laughter is the best medicine", and I'm starting to think that saying was tailor-made for FIFO life and people trying to come terms with having cancer.

During the day, the guys at work kept me howling with their stories and filthy jokes. In the evenings, Jayde kept the laughs going with her sharp observations and general ridiculousness. Between all that and a healthy pay packet, life felt pretty bloody golden.

Sure, I had cancer. But for the first time in a long time, I wasn't worried about it. Could life get better? Possibly. (But let's face it – I wasn't going to push my luck just yet.)

Event 3

You know how people say, *"I was just thinking about so-and-so, and boom – they messaged me!"*? Happens to everyone, right? One minute you're reminiscing, the next they're in your inbox like they've been hiding in your wardrobe.

Well, that exact freaky bit of life-timing happened to me.

It was my first R&R break after becoming mates with Jayde, the walking buddy and housekeeper extraordinaire whose smile had reminded me a lot of someone very special from my past: **Nikki**. Naturally, thoughts of Nikki had been surfacing a lot.

I was at home, working at my iMac in the front bedroom – which by now had more cables than Bunnings and had been unofficially declared *the office*. Messenger was open. A million tabs were running, half of which I no longer remembered opening, when suddenly:

"Hello, Stranger."

The message popped up like something out of a Hallmark movie. It was from someone named *Nikki T****.*

My first thought? The neighbour two doors down is called Nikki. I'd seen her putting the bins out two days ago. "Stranger?" It felt a bit overdramatic.

I clicked the profile... and the penny dropped.

It wasn't neighbour Nikki! It was Nikki who invaded my thoughts every time Jayde smiled.

Just to avoid any confusion (especially for future readers or lawyers), I've mentioned Nikki T earlier in this story. But right up until *this very moment*, I'd only ever known her as *Nicky*, spelt with a 'c' and a 'y', and by her maiden name. I'd had no idea she'd changed the spelling. A small tweak, but it had hidden her in the online ether for all these years.

In that moment, my life – which was already beginning to feel like it was on the up – suddenly **went stratospheric**. I was bouncing off the walls. I had to calm myself down before replying, lest I type something truly idiotic like "OMGOMGOMG HI!!!"

So I replied.

Then she replied.

Then I replied.

And on it went. And it was magic.

For the next eight months, it was as though I had been plugged into some infinite source of light and joy. The guys I worked with were already hilarious, Jayde kept me giggling on our nightly walks, and now Nikki was back in my life – somehow realer and more present than ever.

We talked constantly. Real-time convos, texting, Messenger. Deep chats. Dumb jokes. Glorious nostalgia. The kind of belly laughs which make your ribs ache and leave you wiping away tears.

The only real interruptions to my joy were the same old suspects: **jab days** and **Dr. W's six-monthly PSA calls**.

Jab days were like Russian roulette. Would I go gloomy? Would I start writing poems in binary? No way to tell until the Lucrin kicked in and flipped whichever mental switch it fancied.

The week before my regular check-ins with Dr. W, I'd stress like I was cramming for exams. PSA blood test looming? Cue sleepless nights and full-blown doom spirals.

What if the PSA had risen? What if it wasn't undetectable anymore?

And then the call would come. "Still undetectable," he'd say, casual as you like. And just like that, I'd go from *Eeyore with a death sentence* to *Larry the Extremely Happy Guy* – whoever Larry is, I wanted his life.

Towards the end of the year, things got even more promising. Andrew – the one who got me my current gig – was jumping ship for a better job up in Broome. "Want to come?" he asked. It was the same roster (week on, week off), but with **more money**, which in mining speak translates to: "You'll be sleeping in a shipping container, but you'll be able to afford air-conditioning in it."

I was in.

Or at least, I *planned* to be in.

I crafted a beautiful three-step strategy:

- **Step one**: Resign my current job. Tick.
- **Step two**: Finish my long-suffering home renovation project. Tick.
- **Step three**: Start the new job in January 2023. No tick.

Turns out, on *January 1st*, the new company changed their hiring policy. From that date on, new workers would only be sourced locally from Broome. FIFO was no longer an option.

Oops. Plot twist. I was staying unemployed.

October 2022, life was so good it felt suspicious. I was exercising twice a day. I was eating clean. I had mates I loved working with. I was laughing constantly. My project at home was nearly done. Nikki was back in my life. Even cancer was behaving itself.

By the end of November, the rug had been yanked from under me with the force of a cartoon trapdoor. Suddenly, my job was gone, my walk buddy was 1,500km away, and the lively crib-room banter was replaced by the sound of me, alone, wondering why I hadn't just stayed put.

The only bright spot left was Nikki.

Unfortunately, she lived on the opposite side of the planet, 8 timezones away, and our chats were limited by the laws of physics, the internet, and common decency surrounding sleep.

Still, through December, she kept me going. She probably didn't know it, but she was the only thread tethering me to the sunlight. Every message, every joke, every memory – weighing more than she could ever realise.

And then, as is tragically tradition for me... I fucked up what I had left in spectacular fashion

January came. So did another jab. And this one came with a full deluxe dose of *Wonky Brain Syndrome*.

In the depths of hormone-fuelled weirdness, I wrote Nikki a long, meandering email which, to me, read like a thoughtful and carefully considered roadmap for my future. To Nikki? Apparently, it read more like a disturbing detour through the mind of someone who'd licked a toad.

I didn't mean to upset her. Never in a million years. I could never intentionally hurt her. I *love* Nikki dearly. Always have. Since the day I met her, she's been carved into my story in permanent ink.

But the damage was done. She didn't reply.

And I haven't heard from her since.

Not a day goes by when I don't regret sending that email.

And if I could, I'd take every single word back. Wrap it up. Unsend. Rewrite. Anything.

Because, truthfully, when I had Nikki back in my life... I felt whole.

Write A Book

As 2023 crept in – quietly, awkwardly, like a houseguest who knows they've overstayed their welcome – I found myself staring down the barrel of a pretty miserable January. Christmas had come and gone with all the joy of a lukewarm cup of tea. I was unemployed, alone, and thoroughly fed up with my own company. Even I was getting sick of me.

I missed the random banter and questionable hygiene standards of my former FIFO colleagues. I missed the long walks and deep conversations with Jayde, who had somehow become a lifeline. Mentally? I was teetering on the edge of that dark place I'd sworn I'd never revisit–the one Nikki had unknowingly kept me from until she vanished like a puff of smoke in a magician's act gone wrong.

With the friendships I'd come to rely on now noticeably absent, I found myself asking the Big Questions: What even is friendship? Why did I care more about some people than I did about others? And why did I keep getting friend requests from men named Barry who had four friends and a profile picture of a fish?

In a rare moment of digital courage (fuelled by a fishbowl full of Shiraz and just a touch of spite), I launched an aggressive Facebook cull. Gone were twenty or so "friends" I hadn't spoken to in years. No hard feelings – it was mutual ghosting at best. The lack of contact was as much my fault as theirs, but if I couldn't even be bothered to scroll past their wedding photos, I didn't see the point in maintaining the illusion of connection.

As I deleted, I found myself staring at some of the faces, searching for actual memories involving both them and me. If we shared an event which genuinely meant something – a festival, a road trip, or even just a blurry night in a pub that ended with fish and chips – they were spared. And that took me down an unexpected rabbit hole.

Since finishing my minor DIY masterpieces – the separated lounge and a kitchen which no longer looked like a flat-pack crime scene – I'd been on the hunt for artwork. Something to brighten the place up. Make it feel like a home, not a halfway house for the emotionally burnt out.

So off I trotted to buy picture frames, feeling very much like a man with a vision. Back home, armed with Photoshop and more nostalgia than was healthy, I made collages – photo mosaics of people who had truly meant something to me over the years. Some pictures I yanked from dusty old albums, others I shamelessly downloaded from Facebook like a low-level identity thief. When I was done, I stood back and admired my handiwork. They were beautiful. Honest. Messy. Like me, but with better lighting.

These frames told stories – dozens of them. Smiling faces of friends who had walked in and out of my life, their memory now immortalised on my walls like a curated museum of emotional whiplash. And yet, I missed the close ones. The daily ones. Nikki. Jayde. Even Charlie, who had, understandably, gone a bit quiet.

My mood began to slide. Slowly at first, like socks on a polished floor, but it gathered speed as the months dragged on. I wasn't quite in depression territory, but I could see the neighbourhood. I'd waved at it from across the street.

Charlie had done more than anyone had any right to do, and I'll be grateful to her for the rest of my days. But people move on. Especially from basket cases like me.

I reached out to Nikki. Briefly. A toe-dip into the freezing pool of awkward digital silence. No reply. Perhaps I'd been blocked, or maybe she'd just ghosted harder than a Victorian séance.

Jayde still sent the occasional message, and they always made me smile. She'd left the site, moved into proper mining – real hard hat, hi-vis stuff – not the glorified room service she was so bloody good at. I was genuinely chuffed for her, and still am whenever she shares her wins.

But life... life just kept plodding on like a bored Labrador. I picked up a bit of "Handy Andy" work – small jobs, enough to stay afloat but not enough to feel alive. Even the DIY mojo had abandoned me. I needed something to chew on, mentally speaking. Something to stop me from spiralling into binge-watching renovation shows and convincing myself I could tile a bathroom blindfolded.

Then I remembered the bucket list. I pulled it out, desperate for inspiration. What had I done, and what was still laughing at me? There it was. Number eleven:

11. Write a book.

Almost a year earlier, Nikki and Kerry had both come out of the woodwork after years of radio silence and casually suggested I write one. They were joking, I think. Or drunk. Possibly both. But it stuck. It was the nudge I needed to bin my original plan of writing a thrilling novel about Cat Navarre, international woman of mystery, and instead start this book.

At the time, I was fired up with the enthusiasm of a man who'd just remembered he owned a gym membership. I smashed out a few chapters. Then, in classic Me fashion, I got distracted, demoralised, and ultimately derailed. I'd been here before – started with gusto, only to end up in a pile of discarded drafts and broken dreams.

Still, I told myself it was time to move forward. Time to stand up, dust myself off, and get back on the horse – or at least near the general vicinity of the horse. I powered up the iMac, gave it a stern look, and got typing.

For a few months, I was glued to that computer like a man chasing clarity in the static. I churned out four chapters, started the fifth, and then... fizzled. I reread what I'd written and instantly decided it was garbage. Absolute tosh.

Of course, that was just my deflated opinion. I should've kept going regardless, slapped it all down, and edited later. But I didn't. I turned the iMac off and walked away, dramatically, like it had insulted my mother.

Then came October 2023. I was offered a FIFO job at a goldmine about 600 kilometres east of Perth – once again, courtesy of Andrew B. I took it. Not for the money

– though my bank account resembled a tumbleweed-strewn ghost town – but because I desperately needed to be around people again. I didn't even care if the people turned out to be weirdos. At least weirdos talk.

Boarding the plane, I wondering what my actual job even was. The interview had been vague – probably because it was with the billionaire owner of the mine, who seemed more interested in his golf handicap than my résumé. I assumed someone had read it and thought, he'll do.

The roster was meant to be one week on, one week off. Classic FIFO lie. It quickly morphed into two weeks on, one off. I didn't argue. I was more concerned with whether I'd have anyone to chat with in this remote corner of nowhere. Luckily, the crew was a mixed bag of legends, and I genuinely enjoyed their company and banter.

Management, though? A total shambles. Picture Lord of the Flies, but with high-vis and diesel fumes. Everyone thought they were in charge. It took me nearly two months to figure out who my actual supervisor was– and even then, I wasn't entirely convinced he knew.

After three months of chaos, I waved the white flag. Resigned, packed up my stuff, and came home – with another batch of photos to add to my wall of fame.

It was January 2024. I'd worked through Christmas and New Year, which was as depressing as it sounds. Statistically, it's one of the riskiest times for mental health, and frankly, I didn't trust myself not to make headlines for all the wrong reasons.

Back home, I dived into another collage project – editing, printing, arranging like a scrapbooker with a deadline. While trawling through Facebook, I stumbled on a photo which made me do a double take. It was a long time friend – Louise G – with her grandson. It wasn't the fact she was a grandmother which shocked me (although it did momentarily break my brain). It was that she wasn't already on any of my boards.

I checked. Every wall, every frame. Nothing. Nada. How had that happened? Louise was a keeper. Sure, we hadn't chatted in a while, but she was one of the real ones. I must've misfiled her during the Great Facebook Purge of 2023.

Mortified, I went back to her profile and downloaded every photo which wasn't blurry, cropped weirdly, or featuring a dodgy filter. I made it up to her the best way I knew how – immortalising her on the newest board. I even sent her a copy. She replied instantly. And just like that, I got my old mate back.

So where does Louise fit in this tale?

Well, Nikki and Kerry lit the spark. But Louise? She's the one who came in, steel-capped boots and all, and kicked me squarely in the backside until I got writing again.

And now, here we are. You're reading this. I finally finished the damn book.

The photos are all framed. The walls are full. I might still be messy, but I'm in the picture now too.

Right. Time for one last story before I wrap this up.
Go grab a coffee – or something stronger – and when

you're ready, I'll begin.

Do you remember me telling you I had a job change around the same time as my first wife embarked on her affair in 1999? If you don't, its all in the chapter "Back in the Car Trade".

Before I left the car trade, my wife and I spent Saturday nights in the company of John E and his then-girlfriend, Kate. We'd head for a pub on the outskirts of town, wallop down more beer than was good for us, and it always ended up being a great night. John and Kate were brilliant company.

When I first rocked up in Bridgend as a nightclub manager, John worked for me as a DJ. Over the years, he moved into pub management, eventually taking over as manager when I abruptly vacated the position at Aston's. A few years later, he bought his first pub, then went on an acquisition spree like a man with a Monopoly addiction. Within months, he had seven pubs under his belt, most of them in Bridgend Town Centre.

Oddly, when we went out on Saturdays, we deliberately avoided his pubs. Saturday night was his sacred time off, and he didn't want to be accosted by staff waving spreadsheets or complaints mid-pint.

One particular Saturday, he mentioned a job proposal. We'd both had a few by then, so he promised to come by the cottage during the week for a proper chat.

Over coffee in my lounge, he asked me to come work for him.

Straight away, I said, "No!" Absolutely not. No way was I going back to running pubs and clubs. That chapter was closed, buried, and had a headstone.

Pub management had been fun back when I was single. It's a great lifestyle if you enjoy chaos and never sleeping. But now, married and supposedly settled, I saw no reason to put temptation right under my nose – even though, at the time, I didn't know my marriage was already wobbling like jelly on a trampoline.

But John didn't give up. He laid it out: stock wasn't matching the takings. Classic bar drama. Money was going into pockets instead of tills. He was convinced staff were stealing from him and he needed someone who could sniff out dishonesty like a bloodhound in a butcher's shop.

He knew I had a talent for catching thieves. When he walked into a bar, staff behaved like it was a royal inspection. But as soon as he left, it was back to the wild west. John couldn't be in seven places at once, and the cracks were widening.

To be fair, neither of us liked firing people without hard evidence. Sure, back then employment law was a bit of a joke – you could sack someone for blinking too loudly – but we both preferred to sleep at night.

I didn't want to go back into the nightlife circus, but I wanted to help my mate. We agreed I'd ask Ellen. If she said yes, I'd do it. I fully expected a veto.

"If John needs help, you should help him," she said. To say I was surprised at her reaction was an understatement.

In hindsight, I should've been suspicious. Me working nights gave her even more time with her mystery man.

328

She wasn't going to argue, was she?

The week before I started, I had a casual nose around the bars I'd be overseeing. Watching from the customer side of the bar is always revealing. Staff get sloppy when they think no one's watching. Most of the pubs, I sized up fast. I already knew who was staying and who was about to have their last shift.

Monroes, though, was a tougher read. I'd only popped in at lunchtime. The young blonde behind the bar was either squeaky clean or a criminal mastermind. She was cheerful, efficient, and – so far as I could tell – not nicking anything. I figured if she was honest, I'd get her onside fast. She'd be my eyes and ears. But Monroes wasn't my first mission.

First up: The Courthouse.

What is it with me and courthouses?

This one, like the pub in Cairns, had once been an actual courthouse. Left derelict for years until John and his business partner Dean, a builder, resurrected it into a swanky pub.

The issue wasn't theft. It was morale. The place had an atmosphere thick enough to bottle. Staff were miserable, and it showed. Customers felt it too, and if customers don't feel relaxed in the ambience, they vote with their feet and find a better place for a swift pint.

Day one, I strolled in an hour before opening. I introduced myself to the staff with just my name, walked straight into the manager's office, and parked myself in the manager's chair. Feet on the desk, door wide open.

Only one staff member knew who I was. She recognised me from years back, knew I was close to John, and wisely kept schtum. Marion watched the scene unfold with a knowing smirk.

Ten minutes later, in walked Michelle, the current manager - for the next 30 seconds at least. Her jaw nearly hit the floor.

"Andy! What are you doing here?"

"I'm the new manager of The Courthouse. Pick up anything personal to you off this desk and get the fuck out. You're fired."

No protests. She grabbed a photo frame and a pen, and left. Probably in tears, but I didn't see. I was too busy putting my feet back on the desk.

The atmosphere lifted instantly. Staff actually smiled. I rang John. He was gobsmacked. Michelle had been all sweetness and light around him, and no one else dared speak up.

He told me to stay put for the week.

The Courthouse ran smoother than a Swiss watch. So what did they need me for? I wandered out to Marion.

"Got a job for me?"

She laughed. "Andy, you're the manager. You tell me what to do."

"Nah. I'm just here to tidy up. You're in charge. Hit me."

She handed me cutlery and serviettes. I wrapped knives and forks while she thanked me for getting rid of the one problem the place had. I believed her. Even during Michelle's reign, Marion was the backbone of the place. I suggested to John that she take over as manager. She declined. Retirement was on the horizon, which is a shame, because Marion would have been the best manager the place ever had.

The next week, I took over at Monroes. As predicted, I won over the young blonde. And yes, she became my eyes, ears, and then some. Louise turned out to be a diamond.

I also inherited an assistant manager, Alex. Solid bloke. Did a great job and was quickly promoted to manage his own pub. Well deserved.

His replacement? Adrian. Not my pick, and about as useful as an ashtray on a motorbike, but I didn't care. I had Louise. She mainly ran the bar, but she was always ready and willing to fill the gaps Adrian left wide open. She was a godsend.

And then, Ellen left me, and my home life collapsed like a flan in a cupboard.

Monroes was stable by then, so I packed up and headed back north.

I closed Monroes one Saturday night in April 2000. Sunday, I packed my life into a car and walked down to the Farmer's Arms – my local. Just ten cottage doors away. As I passed each one, I thought of the neighbours I'd miss.

I was standing at the bar ordering a pint when the door swung open behind me.

"Can't let you go without having a beer with my favourite manager."

Louise.

We'd become real mates. She invited me to her wedding later that year, and visited me up north a couple of years later. We lost touch when I emigrated to Australia and she went off down another career path.

Fast forward to now. Ever since Louise replied to my message about her missing photo on the collage board, we've spoken almost daily. Messaging, video calls, the lot.

Right now, it's 8 p.m. Friday in Wales. It's 4 a.m. Saturday here in Perth, Australia. Louise, in full saint mode, is out on a home care visit. Most of Wales is in the pub or cwtched up (pronounced cutched) on the couch - if you are Welsh, that is. Lou is making sure someone's gran has her meds, her blanket, and a hot cup of tea.

Having just spoken to her between calls, she is aiming to be home by midnight to grab a few hours sleep, and start all over again tomorrow. Her dedication hasn't changed since we worked together. Louise is a modern-day saint in scrubs.

To cut a long story short – which, let's face it, I never do – Lou and I are back to being the mates we once were. Maybe better.

Just a few days into reconnecting, I confessed my problem and told her about the book which had gone to stall mode. In classic Louise fashion, she was sympathetic but didn't coddle me. She demanded to read what I had so far. I emailed it and went to bed.

When I woke, she'd already read it. How she found the time is beyond me.

Her message? Get your arse in gear and finish this book.

She's been my proofreader, cheerleader, and comic relief ever since. Thanks to her, the confidence came back. So did the joy of writing.

She made me laugh until my ribs hurt. I hadn't laughed like that since before Nikki vanished.

Louise put me back on track. I'm pages from finishing now. She's read everything but this chapter. Without her, this book would still be a pile of half-written maybes and joining forces in the cardboard box in the shed next to the leaf blower and the VHS tapes.

Does everything happen for a reason? Whether it was fate, coincidence, or the universe having a quiet word, I don't know. What I do know is this: Louise returned when I needed her most. She pulled me out of the fog, reminded me who I was, and gave this book its heartbeat.

Mission accomplished, Lou. And me?

I finished the damn book.

What's Next?

In the week leading up to Christmas, I had a chat with Dr W. The good news? My PSA was still below 0.02 – or, in the words I now consider sexier than "two-for-one desserts," he said it was "Undetectable."

Once I'd filled him in on my general state of being – "still feeling great, still not sick, still only getting up to pee once in the night if I've had a drink before bed" – he casually suggested we give my lymph nodes a bit of a zap. Just like that. No build-up. No dramatic pause. He said it like he was offering me a complimentary side of fries.

The way he lobbed it into the conversation made it sound less like a pressing medical intervention and more like an optional spa treatment. We ran through a few options and landed on "sometime around April/May" – pencilled in, not panic stations.

This time it's only 24 sessions. A doddle, right? Apparently, because he's just targeting the lymph nodes and leaving the prostate alone (already well-and-truly toasted, thank you very much), the side effects will be far less invasive. He made it sound like a Sunday stroll compared to the last round of radiotherapy, which felt more like a forced march through hell with a broken shoe.

The cancer itself still hasn't made a nuisance of itself. I feel better than I have since *Jurassic Park* was in the cinemas first time around. No mystery symptoms, plenty of energy – despite the fact I've already had enough radiation to power a small lighthouse. Dr W never sounds remotely worried when I speak to him, so I'll keep exercising, eating well, resisting the occasional urge to devour an entire cheesecake one sitting, and not worrying about the cancer.

Louise, ever the wise owl, keeps saying, "Everything happens for a reason." Sometimes I want to throw a pillow at her when she says it – but I also suspect she's right. Barbara reckons the cancer showed up as a kind of cosmic intervention: *"change your lifestyle or cop the consequences"*. Both ideas stuck with me. And they helped guide what's turned into one hell of a personal transformation – otherwise known as the world's most aggressive self-improvement course.

Sure, I could have curled up and waited for the inevitable – and who knows, maybe it would've happened by now. But I didn't. I chose to dig myself out of a hole and start walking a different path – one I'll be walking for the rest of my days.

And here's what I've learned: when a soul-crushing diagnosis falls through your front door like a drunk uncle at Christmas, the biggest weapon in your arsenal is a positive mental attitude.

Negativity will show up in all sorts of costumes. It might be a "well-meaning" friend who tells you about their cousin who didn't make it. Or a relative whose idea of support is staring at you like you're halfway in the coffin. Or maybe it's that colleague who thrives on being a human raincloud. Whatever form it takes – cut it loose. Be ruthless. Be downright brutal. Your peace of mind is not a democracy.

Fill your life with people who lift you up – not the ones quietly waiting for you to trip over your own shoelaces. The good ones don't need to be asked – they'll be the ones already holding your hand, passing the snacks, and cracking dodgy jokes in the waiting room.

I've got my Keepers. Some of them aren't mentioned in this book – not because they're not important, but because the narrative didn't take us there. But they're still tattooed on the walls of my heart (and most of them also appear on my lounge room wall in collage form).

Charlie's still one of them. Even though I don't see her much these days, she'll always be on the list. Jayde still drops in with messages that make me laugh or stop and smile. Nikki – we may not be in touch, but she's never left my heart. I still hope she'll pop up one day and say hello. Louise dragged me out of a writing funk, made me laugh until I nearly herniated, and reminded me what real, no-bullshit friendship looks like. These incredible women, and so many others, have been a huge part of my cancer journey – and my life. I'd take a bullet for any one of them. Preferably a small one. In a non-vital area. But still – a bullet.

If your job is dragging you down, change it. Don't tell yourself it's too hard. It's not. I've had three different jobs while writing this book, and I'm hardly a one-man TED Talk. I've got two arms and two legs, same as most people, and that's about the full extent of my qualifications. A moderately clever monkey could do anything I do. You might earn less, sure – but cut your cloth to fit. The point is: if your job is slowly killing you, quit before it finishes the job.

Get moving. Eat something green that didn't come from a packet. If you don't know how, Google it. YouTube it. I did. I now cook meals which don't try to assassinate me from the inside. I even know what a chickpea is. Healthy food and regular movement won't cure everything, but they do wonders for your mood.

And another thing: stop watching the bloody news. I cut it out completely and still knew when the Queen passed away, when the Duke of Edinburgh died, and that there are wars in the Middle East and Ukraine. The important stuff will reach you whether you like it or not – the rest is just noise designed to keep you stressed and scrolling.

So here's the takeaway: bin the crap. Get rid of the stress. Love the people (and animals) in your life unconditionally. Walk your dog, if you have one – it's surprisingly therapeutic. Listen to music that lifts your spirit. Take on projects which stretch your brain. Don't tell yourself you don't have time. You do.

Before I sign off, I want to wish you luck on your journey. Even though we haven't met, I sincerely hope you find love, laughter and happiness in this beautifully finite thing we call life.

So, what's next for me?

Aside from the radiotherapy encore in April, I'm thinking about moving back to Wales. The hills and valleys are calling me. So are the accents. And the ability to buy decent chips after 10pm.

But wherever I end up, I can promise you one thing: I'm going to live while I'm alive.

337

There'll be plenty of time for sleeping when I'm dead.

Ta ta for now.

Andy xxx

Epilogue

If you're anything like me (and I hope for your sake you're not), you'll have reached the end of this book thinking one of two things:

1. "Well, that was an emotional rollercoaster," or

2. "He's going to milk this for a sequel, isn't he?"

Let me reassure you – I'm not planning a sequel. Unless, of course, Netflix calls. In which case, you'll be able to find me on your screens, played by someone ten years younger and twenty kilos lighter, swanning about like I've never sworn at a microwave or cried at a dog food advert.

But in all seriousness – and I promise to keep it brief because we've had enough of that for one book – writing this story has been like laying all my mismatched socks out on the bed and finally finding the bloody pairs. Messy. Cathartic. Occasionally smelly. But ultimately... worth it.

To those who've featured in these pages – thank you. Even the ones I wanted to throttle. You've shaped this weird, wonderful story of mine.

To you, dear reader: thank you for coming this far. For sticking with me through pubs, paddocks, heartbreak, radiotherapy, and Bunnings sausage sizzles of the soul. I hope you laughed. I hope you felt seen. And I hope, whatever you're facing, you know you're not alone.

Now... go live. Big, loud, messy, unapologetic living. Because there is *still* time, and you are *still* here.

And that, my friend, is everything.

Acknowledgements - The Roll Call Of Legends

Charlie - For being there when I was barely holding myself together with duct tape and sarcasm. Your kindness was loud, even in your silence.

Louise - For kicking me up the arse with the gentleness of a cement mixer, for laughing when I couldn't, and for telling me the truth when I didn't want to hear it. You were the spark which kept this whole thing burning.

Nikki - For the moments that mattered. For what was, what could've been, and what still might be. You were the turning point. More than once.

Jayde - For your messages, your encouragement, and your belief in this scruffy old git. You'll always have a seat at the pub in my heart.

Dr W and the Onco Posse - For keeping me ticking, nuking with style, and never making me feel like a number on a chart. You lot are rockstars in lab coats.

Friends unnamed but not unloved - If you're in my collage, you're in my soul. Even if I've forgotten to mention you, your part in this story is real.

The Reader (yes, YOU) - Whether you read this in bed, in a chemo chair, or hiding from your kids in the loo – thank you. You gave this book a purpose. You made it matter.

And lastly...

Cancer - You sneaky bastard. You showed up uninvited, took a wrecking ball to my life, and tried to steal the plot. But here's the twist – I took the pen back. And I've written the ending myself.

Reader Q&A – You Asked, I Definitely Made Up the Answers

Q: Did all of this really happen?
A: Yes. Unfortunately. I'm not imaginative enough to make it up, and too proud to admit which bits I definitely embellished for dramatic effect.

Q: How are you doing now?
A: Alive. Still cheeky. Slightly radioactive. But all systems go.

Q: Will there be another book?
A: If I survive this one being published without being sued, ghosted or disinherited — maybe. If not, I'll just quietly move back to Wales and live out my days as a semi-retired wisdom dispenser with a dog and a thermos.

Q: What's the secret to staying positive?
A: Coffee. Sarcasm. Music from the 80s. Walking shoes. The occasional ugly cry. And knowing that no matter how bad it gets, there's always someone who gets it — and someone who'll pour you a decent cuppa.

Q: Can I message you if I've been through something similar?
A: Absolutely. Unless you're trying to sell me crypto, in which case I'll pretend to be dead.

About The Author

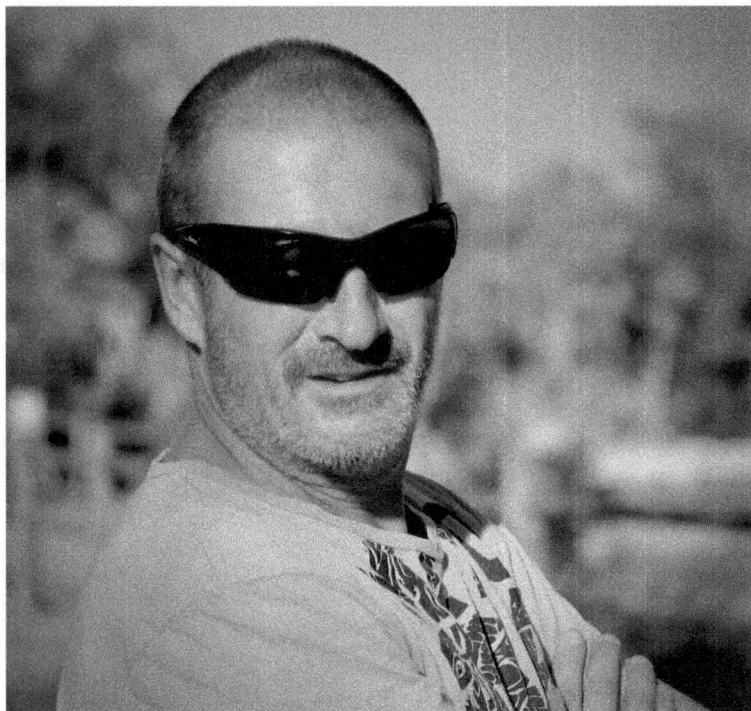

Andy Partington

After decades of colourful careers – including Architectural Technician, Nightclub Manager, Car Salesman, Handyman, FIFO worker and reluctant philosopher – Andy found himself facing the one gig no one applies for: cancer patient. But instead of giving in, he picked up a pen (well, a keyboard), and decided to tell the story.

These days, he splits his time between avoiding bad news, walking for sanity, and ticking off items from his bucket list – with varying degrees of grace and profanity.

He currently lives alone in Two Rocks, Western Australia. Whilst he is the first to admit Australia is an awesome place to live, he is considering the possibility of returning to the place he still considers to be the green, green grass of home, Bridgend, Wales UK.

Diolch am ddarllen y llyfr hwn.

www.ingramcontent.com/pod-product-compliance
Lightning Source LLC
Chambersburg PA
CBHW072133090426
42739CB00013B/3183